THE KETOGENIC DIET

THE ESSENTIAL GUIDE TO START

YOUR KETO LIFESTYLE

EFFORTLESSLY

Table of Contents

Introduction

A healthy way of life is one of life's most respectable & compensating interests. Regardless of whether you need to live more, run farther, or simply look great we're here to offer assistance! Exercise however is just a large portion of the fight. Maybe you've heard the saying that goes "Abs are made in the kitchen?" Well it's totally valid. That is the reason today we need to acquaint you with a diet you may not be familiar with, but rather has prompted some stunning outcomes with regards to weight reduction. One can lose over thirty pounds in the course of six months.

You have most likely heard of the ketogenic diet. This diet has been around for more than nine decades, it has as of late picked up prevalence because of its indicated medical advantages and adequacy in treating an assortment of illnesses, including epilepsy, cancer, & diabetes. The diet is low in carbohydrates and high in fat and works by changing how the body uses and stores its energy.

This book is going to teach you the rudiments to a ketogenic diet, one that is upheld with science and dumbfounding loss of your body fat. We could never embrace something that is only a trend with dull outcomes. This diet utilizes an extraordinary recipe of macro-nutrient intake which manipulates your body to change from utilizing glycogen for energy to utilizing that fuel tank of fat you're bearing.

Chapter1:

What is the Ketogenic Diet?

A ketogenic diet is known very well for being a low carb diet, where the body produces ketones in the liver to be utilized as energy. It has several names such as – keto diet, low carb diet, low carb high fat (LCHF), and so on.

When you eat something high in carbs, your body will create glucose and insulin. Since the glucose is being utilized as an essential energy, your fats are not required and are subsequently put away. Regularly on an ordinary, higher carbohydrate diet, the body will utilize glucose as the principle form of energy. By bringing down the intake of carbs, the body is incited into a state known as ketosis.

Ketosis is a natural procedure the body starts to help us survive when the food intake is low. Amid this state, we produce ketones, which are created from the breakdown of fats in the liver. The true objective of a legitimately kept up keto diet is to compel your body into this metabolic state. We don't do this through starvation of calories yet starvation of carbohydrates.

Our bodies are unfathomably adaptive to what you put into it – when you over-burden it with fats and take away carbs, it will start to consume ketones as the essential energy source. Ideal ketone levels offer numerous health, weight reduction, physical & mental performance benefits.

What Does the Ketogenic Diet Do?

Every different kind of diet has its own specific goals. Most of them simply call for a reduction in overall calories in order for you to lose weight. Cutting down only doesn't always give the best results however. It can be difficult to do and starve your muscles of the nutrients they are craving for.

The ketogenic diet uses the excess of ketones to make your body more dependent on using body fat for fuel. When your body adjusts to the change in carb intake, ketosis begins. The priority fuel for everyday energy shifts from the glucose in carbs towards body fat. After a few weeks on the diet your body will become a fat utilization machine or keto-adapted.

Another way the diet helps you reach your fitness goals is through controlling your blood sugar. Shifting to keto foods and avoiding carbs helps your body stabilize the levels of insulin in your blood stream. This helps you control cravings and keep your metabolism steady. It also encourages fat utilization over glucose fuel.

A Brief History about the Ketogenic Diet

Let's begin with a brief history so that you can know why the ketogenic diet was devised and why it was so popular around a century ago till now. The ketogenic diet was initially planned by Dr. Russell Wilder at the Mayo Clinic to help treat kids with epilepsy seizures. Amid the 1930s, it got extremely well known as a successful approach to treat epilepsy, however as an anti-seizure pharmaceutical turned out to be more predominant amid the 1940s, the ketogenic diet was sheltered (notwithstanding its viability).

In later years, the prevalence of the low carb diet has incited a resurgence of enthusiasm into the ketogenic diet, this time as a very successful technique for getting into shape (specifically, losing fat). Many people have found the ketogenic diet to help them remain sound and fit as a fiddle. Advocates incorporate top athletes like Ben Greenfield and also individuals who have battled with weight issues for quite a while like Jimmy Moore.

The Ketogenic Diet's origins are established in the quest for scientific truth. It is a cure in view of the rule of helping and recuperating, not profiting or making addicts. Continue following the Keto way of life, and show everybody around exactly how intense this diet is!

Chapter 2:

Ketosis: Facts and myths

In the past chapter we talked about the procedure of ketosis and what role it plays in the ketogenic diet. There are a ton of misguided judgments about how ketosis functions, what causes it and what dangers are related with ketosis. In this part we will address a portion of the myths that are regularly expressed about ketosis and additionally particular facts about the procedure.

What is Ketosis?

Ketosis is a typical metabolic process, something your body does to continue working. When it doesn't have enough carbohydrates from foods for your cells to consume for energy, it consumes fat. As a part of this procedure, it makes ketones.

In case you're sound and eating a balanced diet, your body controls how much fat it consumes and you don't typically make or utilize ketones. However, when you cut back on your calories or carbs, your body will change to ketosis for energy. It can likewise occur subsequent to exercising for quite a while and amid pregnancy. For individuals with uncontrolled diabetes, ketosis is an indication of not utilizing enough insulin.

Ketosis can come out to be hazardous when ketones develop. Abnormal levels of ketones prompt lack of hydration and change the chemical of your blood.

What is the Difference Between Ketosis and Ketoacidosis?

Ketosis

When you're on a ketogenic diet, your body will go into a condition of ketosis, which is the metabolic state which happens when your body utilizes ketones as its primary energy source rather than glucose. Amid ketosis, your normally breaks down fat to use as energy as opposed to utilizing carbs for energy (as regularly happens when you eat foods containing carbs). In case you're hoping to burn fat in your body, then ketosis can be something to be thankful for, since it's constraining your body to burn fat as fuel, regularly the fat that you have stored in your body!

Ketoacidosis

Ketoacidosis, on the other hand, is an intense condition that normally happens in type 1 diabetics (and once in a while in end-stage of type 2 diabetics). In ketoacidosis, the body doesn't get enough insulin, which makes the body trust that it's short on glucose – when in fact, there's a great deal of glucose in the blood that can't get into the cells. Therefore, the body begins delivering ketones, which brings about high blood ketone levels in the meantime as high glucose levels.

The Dangers of Ketoacidosis

In the event that you have the type 1 diabetes, one of the genuine difficulties you may face is a condition known as ketoacidosis. The three normal reasons for ketoacidosis are:

Absence of enough insulin. This can happen in case you don't infuse enough insulin or if your insulin needs increment in the light of an ailment, for example, a chilly or seasonal influenza. Blood glucose can't be utilized for energy without enough insulin to help all the while, so the body breaks down fat for energy & high ketone levels result. This can bring about frequent urination, thirst & lack of hydration.

Absence of enough food consumption. In the event that you don't eat enough, your body needs to break down fat for energy, producing high ketone levels. This is especially basic in individuals who are sick & don't have a craving for eating.

Low blood glucose levels. This circumstance can compel your body to break down fat to use as energy, bringing about ketone generation.

Basic Myths about Ketosis

Notwithstanding the scientific confirmation of the advantages that a ketogenic diet can have on one's general wellbeing there is a ton of misconceptions about the means by which keeping to a low carb diet can influence the body, either negatively or positively. In this area we will examine the regular myths about ketosis and how it can influence the body and demystify them. The following are the main 5 myths about the ketogenic diet:

1.   Your body can't work without carbs

At whatever point you ask somebody for what reason they require carbs in their diet, the frequently given answer is "on account of they are fundamental for giving you energy". The word that truly should be accentuated in this sentence is the word fundamental and how this is an immense misguided judgment. The word that ought to be said in this sentence is on the grounds that they are liked to be utilized by the body. The main reason that the body would typically lean toward glucose as its essential fuel, is on the grounds that the grouping of ketone bodies in the fed state are too low to fill in as an optional energy source.

Along these lines once you diminish your carb intake enough, it implies that your body will have the capacity to lower its level of flowing insulin. One of the real functions of insulin is to diminish the level of circling fatty acids, by lessening the movement of hormone-sensitive lipase. What this successfully means is while there is a high coursing level of insulin, your body will never have the capacity to take advantage of its fat stores for energy. When insulin incitement is decreased, the pancreas can discharge the hormone glucagon which initiates lipolysis (unsaturated fat breakdown). The unsaturated fats are then ready to be taken up by the liver and utilized as a part of ketone body synthesis.

2.   **Low starch diets are bad for heart well being**

This is presumably one of the main referred to normal misguided judgments that one can catch wind of taking after a low carb diet. When individuals begin seeing that you eat red meat or add margarine to your vegetables, they believe that is only a formula for heart illness. Individuals' comprehension of this accompanies trusting that eating immersed fat and cholesterol are specifically connected with raising your cholesterol level. This thus is then accepted to be specifically connected to the improvement of cardiovascular infection (CVD).

In actuality, research has it that a low carb diet can truly enhance coronary illness when contrasted with alternate diets. The more carbs you ingest the more the cholesterol your body produces. Cholesterol is a repercussion of glucose digestion. A ketogenic diet has not appeared to have any effects that affect blood tests which demonstrate heart diseases. In this manner a high carb diet is connected to the incendiary heart illness.

3.   **Too much Protein in the Ketogenic Diet Is Bad for Your Kidneys**

This is the greatest myth of them all, in light of the fact that there is positively no confirmation for it, not a solitary review demonstrates that a high-protein, low carb diet harms the kidneys. In case you experience the ill effects of extreme kidney infection by and by, you ought seek after the counsel of your doctor and they may well encourage to limit your protein intake, increment your water intake & increment the intake of different nutrients. Kidney ailment isn't brought about by eating protein.

Low carb diets don't really mean high protein diets. The missing carbs in the low carb diet is supplanted by solid fats. Research has it that individuals who are sound and don't have a past filled with kidney infection can eat some additional protein having no destructive impacts to their kidney or general well-being.

4.   **No one knows the long run effects of eating a low carb diet**

Basically, in what capacity can eating whole foods, solid fats, vegetables, low glycemic fruits, seeds, nuts, berries whole grains be unhealthy? Likewise, individuals who take after a low carb diet discover they have more energy, improved their blood pressure, decrease glucose, and enhanced cholesterol levels. Different advantages that have been noted incorporate better sleep & improved skin quality to give some examples. A straightforward approach to demonstrate this, go to your GP, have your blood work done and then stick to a low carb diet

Nutritional Approach for 6 months and come back to your GP and complete your blood work again and ask him/her whether there has been a change in your general health markers.

5. A Ketogenic Diet Can prompt Osteoporosis

A ketogenic diet is a high fat and moderate protein diet. Having known this now, it's basic to consume proteins to keep up a decent health for your bones. Proteins are one of the essential supplements as far as avoiding osteoporosis is concerned. Additionally a low protein level in one's diet can prompt the deterioration of bone mass and strength.

Bone loss has been attributed to various things including utilization of vegetable oil, inadequacy in magnesium, consuming excessive grain while experiencing gluten intolerance & over-consumption of fructose.

Summary

In summing up, there will dependably be question with respect to the safety and adequacy of a low carb diet, until individuals really comprehend what it implies. By spreading the message and have these sorts of discussions with individuals, ideally we will have the capacity to in the end uproot these normal misinterpretations.

Chapter 3:

Safety check: Is the ketogenic diet right for me?

Since you have a good foundation of the basic knowledge about ketosis and the ketogenic diet you might be prepared to dive in and give it a try. In view of what we have talked about so far, it is improbable that you have anything to lose by trying out the ketogenic diet. In any case, as with any diet there can be a few dangers involved relying upon a number of factors. In this part, we will look at how you can make certain that the ketogenic diet is a safe alternative for you.

Possible Risks Associated with the Ketogenic Diet

In case you're thinking about a high-protein diet, check with your specialist or a nutritionist to check whether it's OK for you. They can help you think of an approach that will ensure you're getting enough fruits, and that you're getting lean protein foods. Keep in mind, weight reduction that lasts is generally in light of changes you can live with for quite a while, not a brief diet. You ought to along these lines converse with your specialist before endeavoring this type of diet as it poses a few dangers which are discussed below.

Low Blood Sugar

At the point when on the ketogenic diet, your body utilizes fat for energy as opposed to its standard fuel, carbs. Toward the starting, your body needs to acclimate to utilizing an alternate fuel source. In case the diet is started too rapidly, or the body is having a troublesome time changing, you can encounter low glucose levels - and the weakness, headaches and other symptoms that come together. This is regularly temporary, and once the body is completely in ketosis, glucose levels stay exceptionally steady and normally lower than normal, as indicated by research.

Acidosis

Ketones are an acid. In this way, when you are in ketosis, your blood can turn out to be more acidic. Nonetheless, the body is great at adjusting and will deliver more bicarbonate to help cradle the acid present in the body. Notwithstanding this, you ought to frequently check blood qualities to guarantee the body is fittingly changing for the expanded acidic condition. Left untreated, acidosis can prompt kidney stones and bone breakdown. Acidosis is simply managed by adding baking soda in water or an assortment of pharmaceutical buffers, all of which should be computed by an expert health specialist for general monitoring & adjustments - meaning you ought to be medicinally checked and shouldn't endeavor to manage it all alone.

Nutrient Deficiencies

Because of the diet limitations, your vitamin and mineral needs are not generally met, making supplementation important, and also optimizing the diet to incorporate supplement rich foods. Utilizing high-fat plant foods, for example, nuts, seeds, avocados & coconut oil in place of animal fats likewise expands vitamin and mineral content while keeping up the vital high fat content. The sorts and measures of supplementation will shift contingent upon the age, sexual orientation, activity level, lab values & level of ketogenic diet started for the person. A dietitian educated in dealing with the ketogenic diet best decides these requirements and will successfully relieve any unfavorable effects to guarantee dietary achievement.

Constipating

This is a typical reaction of the ketogenic diet, yet not usually a hazardous one. The constipation happens in light of the fact that the diet is high in fat and low in fiber, yet this reaction can be avoided with the utilization of medium-chain triglycerides oil & expanded liquid intake. MCT oil is a fat got from coconut and palm oil and is utilized by the body to make ketones. It likewise builds gut transit & in this way eases constipation. Adding high-fiber, low-carb feeds, for example, leafy greens, hemp powder & chia or flaxseed mitigates constipation issues. Stool softeners can likewise be utilized if necessary.

Kidney Stones

Kidney stones, generally called nephrolithiasis, can be a side effect of the ketogenic diet. The basic epilepsy prescriptions topiramate and zonisamide can likewise build the danger of kidney stones. In case the ketogenic diet is started in addition to these pharmaceuticals, the danger of kidney stone formation becomes high. Insufficient liquids can likewise add to kidney stone development. Guaranteeing sufficient hydration & managing acidosis are the two most imperative variables to decline formation of kidney stones. In the last section, we demystified the myth that ketosis would harm one's kidneys; these studies were led on people who had no remarkable health issues. In the event that you battle with kidney issues or liver issues check with your doctor before trying out the ketogenic diet.

Proven Health Benefits of the Ketogenic Diet

Since we have looked at the conceivable threats for some with regards to attempting the ketogenic diet without the correct direction of a health care specialist, let us investigate a portion of the advantages that the ketogenic diet can offer for most. Ideally, this will help you to settle on a choice about whether this is the correct diet plan for you to attempt.

1. Low-Carb Diets Kill Your Appetite (positively)

Hunger is the single most noticeably side effect of dieting. It is one of the fundamental reasons why many individuals feel hopeless and in the end abandon their diets. A best aspect regarding eating low-carb is that it prompts an automated reduction of appetite. The studies reliably demonstrate that when individuals cut carbs and eat more protein and fat, they end up eating much less calories.

2. Low-Carb Diets Lead to More Weight Loss

Cutting carbs is one of the least difficult and best approaches to get more fit. Research demonstrates that individuals on low-carb diets lose more weight, speedier, than individuals on low-fat diets, notwithstanding when the low-fat dieters are effectively confining calories. One reason for this is low-carb diets have a tendency to dispose off excess water from the body. Since they bring down insulin levels, the kidneys begin shedding abundant sodium, prompting quick weight reduction in the first week or two.

In research comparing low-carb & low-fat diets, the low-carbers at times lose 2-3 times as much weight, without being ravenous. Low-carb diets seem, by all accounts, to be especially compelling for up to 6 months, however after that the weight begins cgoing down in light of the fact that individuals abandon the diet and begin eating a similar old stuff.

It is more proper to consider low-carb as a way of life, NOT a diet. The best way to prevail in the long run is to stick to it. Nonetheless, a few people might have the capacity to add healthier carbs after they have achieved their objective weight. Practically no matter what, low-carb diets prompt more weight reduction than the diets they are compared with, particularly in the initial 6 months.

3. Triglycerides have a tendency to go Down

Triglycerides are fat molecules. It is notable that fasting triglycerides, the amount we have of them in the blood after an overnight fast, are a solid heart disease risk factor. Maybe illogically, the primary driver of raised triglycerides is carbohydrate utilization, particularly the basic sugar fructose. At the point when individuals cut carbs, they have a tendency to have a decrease in blood triglycerides. Low-carb diets are extremely powerful at bringing down blood triglycerides, which are fat molecules in the blood and an outstanding danger for heart disease.

4. Increased Levels of HDL (the "good") Cholesterol

HDL and LDL allude to the lipoproteins that carry cholesterol in the blood. While LDL conveys cholesterol from the liver and other parts of the body, HDL conveys cholesterol from the body and to the liver, where it can be reused or excreted. It is known that the higher your levels of HDL, the lower your danger of coronary disease will be.

One of the most ideal approaches to increase your HDL levels is to eat fat and low-carb diets and include much of fat. In this manner, it is not a wonder to see that HDL levels increment drastically on low-carb diets, while they tend to increment just moderately or even go down on low-fat diets. Low-carb diets have a tendency to be high in fat, which prompts an amazing increment in blood levels of HDL, regularly alluded to as the "good" cholesterol.

5. Blood Pressure has a tendency to go down

Having a high blood pressure (hypertension) is an essential risk factor for some ailments. This incorporates coronary disease, stroke, kidney failure among many others. Low-carb diets are a compelling approach to lessen hypertension, which ought to prompt a diminished danger of these maladies and help you live longer. Studies demonstrate that diminishing carbs prompts a huge lessening in hypertension, which ought to prompt a decreased danger of numerous normal ailments.

6. Low-Carb Diets Are Therapeutic For Several Brain Disorders

It is frequently claimed that glucose is vital for the mind and it's valid. Some part of the brain can just burn glucose. That is the reason the liver produces glucose out of protein in the event that we don't eat any carbs. However, an expansive part of the brain can likewise consume ketones, which are formed amid starvation or when carbs intake is low. This is the working behind the ketogenic diet, which has been utilized for quite a long time to treat epilepsy in children who don't react to medication treatment.

7. Reduced Blood Sugar & Insulin Levels, With a Major Improvement in Type 2 Diabetes

The low levels of insulin in the body cause more prominent lipolysis and free-glycerol discharge contrasted with an ordinary diet when insulin is around 80-120. Insulin has a lipolysis-blocking impact, which can restrain the utilization of unsaturated fats as energy. Additionally, when insulin is brought to low levels, gainful hormones are discharged in the body, for example, growth hormone & other effective growth hormones. In this manner the most ideal approach to lower glucose and insulin levels is to decrease carbohydrates utilization. This is additionally an extremely compelling approach to treat and conceivably even reverse the type II diabetes.

In summary, the ketogenic diet is a high fat, low carb diet that has useful impacts of fat and weight reduction, enhanced satiety, improved metabolic syndrome & decreased inflammation. The diet is at the front line of the reanalysis of the relationship between dietary fat, carbs & heart diseases. It likewise has effects beneficial to athletic performance, mental clarity, & the Alzheimer's disease. It can be a trying diet to keep up with, it can be related with micro-nutrient deficiencies, it can be unsafe in diabetics, and it might have a problematic "transition stage" as one progresses toward becoming keto-versatile. In any case, for the perfect individual, it can have a significant positive effect.

Chapter 4:

The 3 basic principles of a ketogenic diet plan

With all the useful information that you have learnt about ketogenic diet until now, it might appear that taking after the diet itself is considerably more complicated. In any case, this is a long way from the case. So as to effectively consolidate the ketogenic diet into your way of life, there are just a couple of essential rules that you need to take after. When you adhere to the 3 fundamental standards of a ketogenic diet plan, you will have the capacity to effortlessly make the ketogenic diet some portion of your life. The accompanying rules are the place to begin when arranging your ketogenic diet plan. You should monitor your sustenance intake so as to accomplish full ketosis. As you get more fit, you will likewise need to reevaluate what you are eating. The correct measures of each macro-nutrient you require for your body to go into the ketosis state will vary from individual to individual. With a specific end goal to help you get into the general ketosis ballpark, here are a few suggestions from specialists.

Low carb

Different to the conception that many people have about the ketogenic diet, the diet includes some sugar utilization. The key is that the measure of sugars that you are eating must be constrained for ketosis to start so you can encounter the advantages of the diet, which start so you can encounter the advantages of the diet, which start with that metabolic process. For your carb amount, the aggregate amount must be at least less than 100g every day and for many people less than 50g. What's more, for individuals with insulin sensitivities, you may need to use less than 30g or 20g every day. For genuine athletes, the sugar amount may be higher based upon your level of training.

Higher Fat

You will eat significantly more fat on this diet and this may startle a few people at first. Things being what they are there is very little amount as the quality of the fat that you consume. Trans-fatty fats are one of the unhealthiest substances in our foods today and are available in many processed foods. These fats are absolutely poisonous and give little of the food the body needs. What we have to comprehend is that fat now is being utilized as a fuel for our bodies rather than as reinforcement. In case the glucose runs out-you will require more fat to replace the carbs that you have avoided. In the wake of restricting starches and eating a moderate measure of protein, whatever is left of what you eat ought to be healthy fats like ghee, coconut oil, olive oil, avocado oil, and creature fats. However, that means you end up eating a considerable amount of fat!

Moderate Protein

Low carb diets like the Atkins Diet permit you to eat as much fat and proteins you need. The hypothesis is that since fat and protein are so filling, you will consequently eat less. This is not as per genuine ketogenic standards since eating excessively protein can meddle with accomplishing ketogenesis. To calculate the minimum and maximum protein intake in order to remain in ketosis, you ought to multiply your weight (measured in lbs) by 0.6 and 1.0 to get the least and most of protein in grams you ought to eat every day.

The three fundamental types of keto diets

There are three essential varieties of keto diet-standard keto dieting (SKD), cyclical keto dieting (CKD), and targeted keto dieting (TKD). The kind of diet you utilize will depend on trial and error & your goals.

- Standard Keto Dieting-This is the most basic, fundamental variety of keto dieting. SKD does not have time of starch re-feeding like CKD and TKD do. This is essentially a diet that has a static ketogenic diet nutrient intake (moderate protein, high fat and low sugar).
- Cyclical Keto Dieting-This type of keto dieting actualizes recurring sugar re-feeds to help reestablish muscle glycogen stores for a brief

timeframe after stores have been totally exhausted. The time span between carbs loads will shift based on the client inclination and their training intensity & objectives.

- Targeted Keto Dieting-The last type of keto dieting, TKD, uses discontinuous periods of starch intake particularly around the exercise time period. The objective here is to give enough glucose to upgrade athletic performance without repressing ketosis for long timeframes.

What to Eat While On the Ketogenic Diet

While you may have numerous alternatives as far as what to eat when you are adhering to the rules of the ketogenic diet, there are a couple of foods that you will do well to avoid all together. These foods offer no nutritious esteem, and specifically contradict the aims of the ketogenic diet. In this section, we will talk about a couple of foods that you ought to attempt your best to avoid with a specific end goal to receive the most benefit from following the ketogenic diet. We will likewise look at the sort of foods that it is alright for you to eat every now and then, and those which you can eat as much as you need.

Foods to Avoid

Going on a ketogenic diet can be exceptionally troublesome in the earliest stages. Comprehending what to eat and what not to eat sets aside some opportunity to get used to, so in case you commit a few errors at the beginning don't be too hard on yourself. It's ideal to commit an error and gain from it than to commit an error and not understand it was in mistake. There's continually going to be foods that are awful for us with regards to eating. In case you're as yet uncertain about any items or nourishments that won't be keto-friendly, don't stress yourself. Here, you'll discover a list of things that you ought to dependably be watchful for.

- Sugar. It's ordinarily found in soda, juice, sports drinks, candy, chocolate, and frozen yogurt. Anything that is processed and sweet you can consider in all probability contains sugar. Keep away from sugar no matter what.

- Grains. Any wheat items (bread or buns), pasta, grain, cakes, cakes, rice, corn, and beer ought to be avoided. This incorporates entire grains like wheat, rye, grain, buckwheat, & quinoa.

- Starch. Keep away from vegetables (like potatoes and yams) and different things like oats, muesli, and so on. Some root vegetables are alright with some restraint.

- Trans Fats. Margarine or whatever other spreadable substitution margarine ought to be kept away from as they contain hydrogenated fats (terrible for us).

- Fruit. Stay away from any large fruits (apples, oranges, bananas) as they're amazingly high in sugar. A few berries can be consumed with some restraint.

- Low-fat foods. These have a tendency to be substantially higher in carbs and sugar than full-fat variants. Ensure you read the package to ensure an oversight isn't made.

- Milk. This is off the list since it contains a considerable measure of lactose, a type of sugar, which makes it high in starches. Low-and reduced fat dairy items are to be avoided as they're excessively processed, which strips out supplements like the fatty acids that make you feel full.

- Soft drinks. These are loaded with an excessive amount of sugar or potential carbs to be permitted in case you're serious about keto. A few people will drink diet, or "zero," soft drinks, however avoid them in case you can in light of the fact that the citrus extract and aspartame frequently found in them may wreck your trip to ketosis.

- Refined fats and oils like sunflower, canola, soybean, grape seed, and corn oils, which have been processed at high temperatures, making free radicals that can harm cells.

- Factory-cultivated animal products & sea foods, which are lower in nutrients and regularly more harmful for the environment than their healthier partners; and processed hotdogs and sausage, which, as a general rule, have additives called nitrates that have been linked to disease.

- Processed foods. These incorporate sustenances that incorporates preservatives and additives, for example, carrageenan, monosodium glutamate (MSG), sulfites, Bisphenol A (BPA) and wheat gluten.

Foods to Eat Occasionally

At this point, you ought to have a truly good idea of what to eat on a ketogenic diet. Ensure that you read and re-read through the list of acceptable foods to build a mental picture around what kind of meals you will need to eat. The limit that you should adhere to with regards to these foods is based altogether in light of your individual carb limit, which obviously will be dictated by your body needs and your general goals. Here is a concise list of a portion of the foods you ought to eat.

- Eggs. Eggs are one of the healthiest and most flexible foods on the planet. One egg contains under 1 gram of carbs and less than 6 grams of protein, making eggs a perfect sustenance for a ketogenic way of life. Also, eggs have been proved to trigger hormones that accelerate feelings of being full and keep glucose levels steady, prompting lower calorie intakes for up to 24 hours. It's imperative to eat the whole egg, as the greater part of an egg's nutrients are found in the yolk. This incorporates the cell antioxidants lutein & zeaxanthin, which help secure eye health.
- Coconut oil. This has one of unique properties that make it appropriate for a ketogenic diet. In the first place, it contains medium-chain triglycerides (MCTs). Unlike long-chain fats, MCTs are taken up specifically by the liver and changed over into ketones or utilized as a quick source of energy. Truth be told, coconut oil has been utilized to build ketone levels in individuals with Alzheimer's infection and different issue of the brain and sensory system. The primary fatty acids in coconut oil are lauric acid, a marginally longer-chain fat. It has been recommended that coconut

oil's blend of MCTs and lauric acid may promote a sustained level of ketosis

- Nuts and seeds. These are healthy, high-fat and low-carb nourishments. Frequent nut utilization has been connected to a lessened danger of heart diseases, certain cancers, depression among other diseases. Moreover, nuts and seeds are high in fiber, which can help you feel full and retain fewer calories finally. Albeit all nuts and seeds are low in net carbs, the amount changes a bit among the distinctive types.
- Low-Carb Vegetables. Non-starch vegetables are low in calories and carbs, however high in numerous nutrients, including vitamin C and a few minerals. Vegetables and different plants contain fiber, which your body doesn't process and assimilate like different carbs.
- Fermented Soy Products. In the event that you enjoy soy items, which are not prescribed because of the many negative health impacts related with soy, you ought to just use non-genetically modified soy items which have been fermented.

Conclusion

A ketogenic diet doesn't should be agonizing. Truth be told, it can be useful to your way of life if done appropriately. As a rule, a ketogenic diet will give all the nutrients that you need. Make sure to follow this thorough list if at all you are on a ketogenic diet to make sure that you get the best possible nutrients you require while in ketosis.

The Matter of Substitutes

With a large portion of the nourishments that you are likely usual to eating consistently at present are not permitted as a component of a strict ketogenic diet. Does this imply you will never again have the capacity to appreciate the essence of your most loved sustenances? This is not really the situation. There are numerous alternatives with regards to substituting your most loved nourishments and fixings with ketogenic diet friendly sustenances. In this part, we will look at what nourishments or meals you can use to supplant with those high carbs favorites.

Breakfast

For your most loved breakfast foods, there are loads of low carb alternatives that are quite recently scrumptious, if not more so. Try switching flavored yogurt with full fat Greek yogurt or coconut milk yogurt. You can likewise take a stab at having full fat curds or sour cream. For added flavor, blend in a couple of toasted nuts, berries or your most loved flavors.

For your most loved breakfast cereal, substitute chia pudding, flax granola or toasted nuts. You can likewise have a go at eating salted caramel pork skin oat, or blended nuts that have been toasted so that they are pounded and firm.

With regards to cereal, an awesome substitution can be chia seed oats or flaxseed oats. Pancakes & waffles can be made with various elements for a lower starch form. For instance attempt cream cheddar pancakes or almond flour waffles!

Dinner

For those supper dinners that are stacked with starches, there are low sugars choices also. For instance, rather than having a burger and French fries, have a medium estimated steak with spread on it and broccoli as an afterthought. In the event that steak is not your thing, or a tad bit aspiring for your budget, attempt a burger without a bun or utilize vegetables for buns.

For pizza, have a pizza with an alternative crust. One case of this is a crust made with almond flour. You can add cheddar to the crust for a tad bit of additional indulgence, and you won't know the distinction when contrasted with a customary pizza crust.

Fried chicken is another solace sustenance that can be made similarly as great, with low carbs alternatives. Take a stab at utilizing pork rinds that have been ground up in a sustenance processor and adding parmesan cheddar to it. This will give you the fried chicken you adore, with a fresh crust and a moist & delicious inside.

For your most loved canned soup, make soups yourself utilizing crisp ingredients, including fresh cream as a base. Take a stab at making your most loved soup in mass and freezing it for fast and simple dinners when you require them. In order to replace your most loved pasta, which is a lethal food as far as the ketogenic diet is concerned, which means it is completely jam packed with carbs, why not attempt zoodles? These are zoodles made of zucchini which you can cover with your most loved cream sauce.

The Most Famous Diet in History

Since we have already covered the essentials concerning the ketogenic diet, let us additionally go over what a few people consider the most popular ketogenic diet ever-the Atkins Diet. The Atkins diet is a low-sugar diet, for the most part suggested for weight reduction. Defenders of this diet guarantee that you can shed pounds eating as much protein and fat as you need, provided that you avoid foods that are high in carbs. In the previous 12 years, more than 20 studies have demonstrated that low-carb diets are compelling for weight reduction, and can prompt different health improvements.

The diet was initially viewed as unhealthy and slandered by the standard health experts, for the most part because of the high saturated fat it contains. However, new reviews have demonstrated that saturated fat is safe. From that point forward, the diet has been considered altogether and appeared to prompt more weight reduction than low-fat diets, and more prominent changes in glucose, HDL (the "great" cholesterol), triglycerides & other health markers.

In spite of being high in fat, it doesn't raise LDL (the "bad") cholesterol on average, in spite of the fact that this happens in a subset of people. The Atkins diet is divided into 4 unique stages:

1.	Phase 1 (Induction): Under 20 grams of carbs every day for 2 weeks. Eat high-fat, high-protein, with low-carb vegetables like verdant greens. This initiates the weight reduction.

2.	Phase 2 (Balancing): Slowly include more nuts, low-carb vegetables and little measures of fruits back to your diet.

3.	Phase 3 (Fine-Tuning): When you are near your objective weight, add more carbs to your diet until weight reduction backs off.

4.	Phase 4 (Maintenance): Here you can eat the greatest number of healthy carbs as your body can endure without recapturing weight.

These stages however are somewhat convoluted and may not be not fundamental. You ought to have the capacity to get in shape and keep it off provided that you adhere to the meals plan we studied before. A few people avoid the induction stage & incorporate a lot of vegetables and fruits from the begining. This approach can be exceptionally successful also. Others want to simply remain in the induction stage inconclusively. This is otherwise called a low-carb ketogenic diet (keto). It is in reality simple to follow the Atkins diet at most of the eateries.

- Get additional vegetables rather than bread, potatoes or rice.
- Order a supper based on fatty meat or fatty fish.
- Get some additional sauce, margarine or olive oil with your meal.

Isn't The Ketogenic Diet The Same As The Atkins Diet?

Not so much (it will depend on how you translate the Atkins diet and what you eat on it):

1. The Atkins Diet is a Low Carb Diet

Many individuals translate the Atkins diet to be a low sugar diet, and when you attempt the Atkins diet, that is the manner by which you comprehended it. You will check the grams of sugars you eat however don't generally focus on the protein or fat amounts.

A few people replace the starches they would some way or another be eating with more lean meat in their diet (accordingly expanding the protein intake however not the fat intake). Also, sadly, eating excessively protein is one thing that can keep your body from getting into ketosis (which is the primary advantage of a ketogenic diet). Obviously, in case you think Atkins represents a high fat diet, then what you think about the Atkins diet could be significantly nearer to the ketogenic diet.

2. The Atkins Diet Doesn't Require Ketone Testing

As a rule, the vast majority on the Atkins diet don't do ketone testing to ensure they're in ketosis whereas that is a major some portion of the ketogenic diet (in light of the fact that being in ketosis is such a significant part of the ketogenic diet). Many individuals however do call the more present day type of a ketogenic diet a Modified Atkins Diet.

A strict ketogenic diet can be contrasted with the induction phase of the Atkins Diet. All in all, which one is the better choice? The straightforward truth is that both diets will work to some degree however in case you need to quick track your prosperity, you should watch what you eat.

Chapter 5:

Some side Effects to Expect with the ketogenic diet

Like any change to your diet, when beginning a ketogenic diet, it is typical to experience at least one side effects as the body adjusts to another method for eating. While going on a ketogenic diet, the body needs to switch its fuel source from the glucose in carbs to utilizing its own particular fat stores, and this can prompt encountering some side effects.

Despite the fact that the antagonistic impacts identified with the ketogenic diet are less severe than those of anticonvulsant pharmaceuticals used to treat epilepsy, people taking after the diet may encounter various undesirable impacts. Before we take a gander at the side effects related with ketogenic diet it's imperative to know whether or not you are in ketosis. How would you know you're in ketosis? It's possible to quantify it by testing urine, blood or breath tests. In any case, there are likewise obvious side effects that require no testing like:

- Dry mouth and extended thirst. Unless you drink enough and get enough electrolytes, for example salt, you may feel a dry mouth. Attempt some bouillon or two daily, in addition to as much water as you need.

- Increased urination – another ketone body, acetoacetate, can end up in the pee. This makes it possible to test for ketosis utilizing urine strips. It likewise can bring about going to the lavatory more frequently. This is the primary driver of the increased thirst.

- Keto breath – this is because of a ketone body called CH3)2CO getting away by means of our breath. It can make a man's breath smell "fruity", or like nail polish remover. This odor can once in a while likewise be felt from sweat, when working out. It's regularly temporary.

How Do You Measure Ketosis?

There are three approaches to quantify for ketones, which all accompany advantages and disadvantages:

1. Urine strips
2. Breath ketone analyzers
3. Blood ketone meter

Urine strips

Urine strips is the most basic and cheap approach to measure ketosis. It is the main alternative for generally learners. You plunge the stick in your pee, and after 15 seconds the color change will disclose to you the presence of ketones. In case you get a high reading (a dull purple color) you'll realize that you're in ketosis.

Pro: Ketone strips are accessible in consistent drug stores and they're extremely cheap. An emphatically positive test dependably demonstrates that you're in ketosis.

Con: Results can vary contingent upon how much fluid you drink.

The strips don't demonstrate an exact ketone level. At long last and in particular, as you turn out to be progressively keto-adjusted and your body reabsorbs ketones from the urine, urine strips may end up being untrustworthy regardless of the possibility that you're in ketosis. Along these lines the test may sometimes stop working – continually demonstrating a negative outcome – when you've been in ketosis for half a month.

Breath ketone analyzers

Breath ketone analyzers are a basic approach to measure ketones in your breath. They are more costly than urine strips. However, they are less expensive than blood ketone meters over the long run, since they are reusable a number of times. These analyzers don't give you an exact ketone level, yet rather a color code for the general level. Research shows that there is better than average relation with blood ketones in many situations.

Pro: Reusable, basic test.

Con: Does not generally relate well with blood ketones. Not exact, and can sometimes show misleading.

They are more costly than urine strips than blood meter.

Not compact, needs PC hookup to read.

Blood ketone meters

Blood ketone meters show a correct and current level of ketones in your blood. They are at present the best quality level and the most correct approach to measure your ketosis level. The significant disadvantage, in any case, is that they are very costly.

Pro: Exact and reliable.

Con: Expensive since it requires pricking your finger for a drop of blood.

What Should Your Ketone Levels Be?

This ends up being a somewhat entangled question to reply. The ideal ketone levels for you will depend a great deal on what your objectives are for being on a ketogenic diet. In case it's weight reduction, then your ketone levels can be much lower than somebody who is doing keto for growth or epilepsy treatment.

Who Shouldn't Go On A Ketogenic Diet?

While sugars are not basic for our bodies, there are a few people for whom a ketogenic diet isn't perfect.

1. Type 1 Diabetics
2. Type 2 Diabetics utilizing Insulin
3. Women who are breastfeeding
4. People on specific medicines e.g., for hypertension

In the event that you can be categorized as one of those classes, then please make a special effort to be extra careful while attempting a ketogenic diet. The ketogenic diet is a device, however that doesn't mean it ought to be utilized constantly and by everybody. We exceedingly propose running restorative tests to guarantee you don't have any basic health conditions before you begin any kind of diet or exercise program. Low carb diet side effects are manageable in the event that you comprehend why they happen and how to limit them. Understanding your physical responses will help you avoid the most awful of the side effects, and shield you from stopping before you escape the chute. Following half a month, these symptoms will die down as you move toward becoming "keto-adjusted" and ready to consume fat rather than glucose for fuel. The list below incorporates the most well-known low carb diet side effects, and furthermore tips on the best way to deal with them.

Frequent Urination

After the first day or so, you'll see that you are in the lavatory urinating more frequently. Your body is burning up the additional glycogen (stored glucose) in your liver & muscles. Breaking down glycogen discharges a considerable measure of water. As your carb intake and glycogen stores drop, your kidneys will begin dumping this abundant water. What's more, as your circling insulin levels drop, your kidneys begin discharging abundant sodium, which will likewise bring about more incessant urination.

Hypoglycemia (Low Blood Sugar)

In the event that you've been eating a higher carb diet, your body is accustomed to putting out a specific measure of insulin to deal with the sugar which gets made from that whole carb consumption. When you all of a sudden drop your carb intake on a ketogenic diet plan, you may have some transient low glucose scenes that will feel exceptionally alarming.

Headaches

While your body is adjusting to ketosis, headaches can show for different reasons. You may likewise feel somewhat bleary eyed, and may encounter some influenza like side effects for a couple days. It's typically a mineral issue. To check whether it's sodium loss, take a stab at putting a quarter teaspoon of salt in a glass of water and drink it. You ought to feel better in around 20 minutes.

Finally, it's vital towards the beginning of the diet to increase your salt and water intake. It will improve following 3-4 days. In case it doesn't, add some more carb to your day by day total. This is one of those low carb diet symptoms for which there is no strong clarification, and it appears to differ by individual.

Constipation

This is another most widely recognized low carb diet symptoms, and is typically a component of lack of hydration, salt loss, eating excessive dairy or an excessive number of nuts, or perhaps magnesium irregular imbalances. In the event that 400 mg of magnesium citrate isn't helping, you might need to decrease your dairy item utilization to rebalance your calcium intake to your magnesium consumption, drink more water or cut back on the measure of nuts you are eating.

Sugar Cravings

As your body experiences the way toward retrofitting itself to consume fat rather than sugar, there's a two to 21 day transit period where carb desires will be more terrible. Attempt a portion of the tips on the most proficient method to stop sugar longings. In case you can endure it, the longings will die down and in the long run vanish, provided that you don't swindle. Eating a lot of carb will bring the desires back, and for a few of us, eating sugar in any amount will begin the slide down that tricky slant to carb over-burden.

Diarrhea

This low carb diet reaction is not strange, and ought to reveal itself over a couple days. It can happen in light of the change in diet, or if a rash choice is made as far as possible fat intake on a low carb diet, which brings about eating excessive protein.

To treat, attempt a teaspoon dosage of sugar free Metamucil or plain psyllium husk powder just before you eat. The fiber will ingest the overabundant water in the colon and ought to help settle loose stools.

Unsteadiness or Weakness

This is a symptom of hypoglycemia or low glucose. It could likewise be a side effect of low mineral levels. Add some more protein to your day by day diet to counterbalance the drop in glucose levels, and eat more salt (put a 1/4 teaspoon of salt in a glass of water and drink it) and incorporate more potassium containing foods. You could likewise take 1-3 potassium citrate supplements of 99 mg, however not more than that. It's ideal to get potassium from food. Taking excessively numerous potassium supplements can stop your heart, so do some selection.

Sleep Disturbances

A few people report that they can't stay asleep when on a ketogenic diet. This might be an indication that insulin and serotonin are low. Attempt this plan: eat a snack that contains both protein & some starch just before bed. The sugar will build insulin, which will permit more tryptophan from the protein to get into the brain.

Kidney Stones

A few people will bring this symptom up when they are attempting to persuade individuals that low carb diet reactions are risky. They construct this in light of the reports of higher rates of calcium based kidney stones revealed by doctors who direct ketogenic diets for kids with epilepsy. Yet, this is not an exact comparison.

Hair loss

A few people report that they encounter quickened baldness when on a low carb or ketogenic diet. This situation is not related entirely to a ketogenic diet, but rather is more probable related with any significant change in diet.

Bad breath

This is typically temporary and it will probably vanish following fourteen days without coming out of ketosis by reintroducing carbs. On the off chance that bad breath is an issue, minty without sugar gum or breath freshener can help veil the odor. Another arrangement is to consider additional thorough oral cleanliness by brushing teeth and utilizing mouthwash all the time as the day progresses.

Should You Go On A Ketogenic Diet?

Likewise with any diet or work out regime, it's an individual decision. The expert's take is that a ketogenic diet could be extraordinary on the off chance that you currently have your body and health basically sort out.

This means you've officially done lab testing to ensure you don't have health conditions like adrenal exhaustion, thyroid issues, vitamin or mineral insufficiencies, or parasites or other gut pathogens. Since in the event that you do have any of these issues (or others), it's very likely that a ketogenic diet could simply put more weight on your body and maybe even worsen some of these issues.

What's more, in the event that you do attempt a ketogenic diet, recall that the essential precepts of a Paleo diet still apply i.e., ensure you eat heaps of supplement thick foods and those low in toxins. A ketogenic diet, like other dietary mediations, has advantages and disadvantages. People who have hidden conditions that put them at risk for different ailments are more susceptible to getting side effects related with dietary changes. Basically real dietary changes ought to be made under the correct direction by specialists, even in normal people, however most particularly in those with prior medicinal conditions.

Along these lines, there you are. In case you get ready for them, these low carb diet symptoms can be minor barriers, and after you acclimate to the diet, they ought to show signs of improvement and lastly die down. From that point onward, you should feel really darned good.

Chapter 6:

Do I need to calorie count?

Presently this is presumably not what you need to hear but rather yes, you should do some calorie counting. It is fundamental science-in case you need to get fit; you have to ensure that you utilize more energy than you take in daily. The good news is that this calorie counting won't feel prohibitive as it would in typical diets and that there is some extension for playing with the figures.

The meaning of a calorie

A calorie is the measure of energy required to raise the temperature of 1 gram of water by 1 degree Celsius. The calories in foods are truly kilocalories or 1000 calories. When we say that a starch like sugar has 4 calories for every gram, we truly imply that it has 4 kilocalories for each gram. This implies that 1 gram of sugar has adequate energy to raise the temperature of one thousand grams of water by four degrees Celsius. The calories in foods actually give a measure of the energy content of the food.

Calories are the energy in food. Your body has a steady demand for energy and utilizes the calories from food to continue working. Energy from calories fuels each of your activity, from squirming to marathon running.

What number of calories does your body burn?

The quantity of calories that you require relies on upon the size of your body and your level of activity. A large individual requires a bigger number of calories than a small individual, an active individual requires a greater number of calories than an inactive individual, and men require a larger number of calories than ladies. The base measure of energy required when resting, called the Basal Metabolic Rate (BMR) can be computed utilizing the Mifflin-St Jeor equations. These equations require the weight in kilograms, the height in centimeters, and the age in years. The BMR must be multiplied by an activity factor to assess the day by day calorie necessities. The following equation can give a gauge of your day by day caloric requirement:

Male: BMR = 10×weight + 6.25×height - 5×age + 5

Female: BMR = 10×weight + 6.25×height - 5×age – 161

Setting a Target Body Weight

When you have figured your present calorie requirements, you need to calculate the calorie necessities for the body that you might want to have. Your objective weight ought to be to such an extent that your Body Mass Index falls between the typical scope of 18.5 to 24.9. For instance, in case you are a 35-year old, lightly-active female with a height of 5 feet, 6 inches and a weight of 160 pounds, you require 1,978 calories for every day to keep up your weight.

Determining the Calories in Food

When you know what number of calories you have to accomplish your objective weight, you need to determine what number of calories is in the food that you eat. The table below demonstrates the calories of sugars, proteins, fats, & alcohol. Fiber comprises of sugars that are not absorbable and can be subtracted from the amount of aggregate carbs.

Carbohydrates	4 Calories per gram
Proteins	4 Calories per gram
Fats	9 Calories per gram
Alcohol	7 Calories per gram

Set up a base line

In case you are not used to dieting & measuring food, the most ideal approach to begin is to simply eat normally for around one week, yet weigh

& measure everything that you eat or drink. This will build up a base line of your ordinary dietary patterns & your caloric intake.

For instance, let us say that you might want to eat some sunflower seeds. The nutrition level says that one serving comprises of one ounce or 28 grams, and that the one-pound bundle has 16 servings. This 28-gram serving has 190 calories. Get a handful that contains all the sunflower seeds which you will eat, & prior to eating a single piece, weigh them. Assume that they weigh 30 grams. You know that there are 190 calories in 28 grams, so you calculate:

One handful = 30 grams × (190 calories/28 grams) = 204 calories

You write this in your diary and after that you can enjoy your seeds.

Once your diet begins

You will need to know what number of grams of food has a particular number of calories. In the event that you need to eat just 100 calories of sunflower seeds, what number of grams would it be a good idea for you to eat? Because you are aware that twenty eight grams contain one hundred and ninety calories, you can calculate:

Weight required = 100 calories × (28 grams/190 calories) = 14.7 grams

Round this figure to 15 grams, weigh that measure of seeds, write it in your diary, and enjoy realizing that you are eating just 50% of your previous calories. You may even now feel hungry, however such is reality. You need to sacrifice for what you need. You won't starve.

The initial few days of monitoring your calories are the hardest on the grounds that you need to look into the quantity of calories of each new food. It might appear that you are investing more time recording what you eat than eating. However do not be demoralized.

Counting calories is valuable at the start for educational purposes. Many individuals who endeavor a ketogenic (low carb high fat) diet end up really consuming a low carb high protein diet. It can be truly hard to get the fat content of your meals up to the correct level. This is the reason calorie counting is essential – it is a reality checking on your macronutrient proportions and you can modify your meals according (I.e. pump up the fat content by including a specific measure of butter or oil.) As you begin to get lose weight, it's additionally critical in light of the fact that you will take in your "sweet spot" for weight reduction – many individuals find that below a specific calorie edge they have decreasing weight reduction returns.

You have to go for a day by day calorie deficit of 500 calories so as to lose about a pound in a week. Try not to go and cut the calories too drastically in the expectation of losing more- cutting 500 is bounty when you consolidate it with the enhanced fat-burning capacity of your body on this new plan.

With a ketogenic diet it is essential to keep the proportion of macronutrients ideal, notwithstanding observing your general calorie count so it pays to either search for an application that empowers you to check what the calorie count of the food that you need to eat is.

All in all, this diet is more lenient than most in the event that you do surpass your calorie count once in a while, provided that the sustenance is low in carbs.

Calorie counting here is somewhat irritating first yet will pay awesome profits at last. In the end, once you get used to eating along these lines and what the portion sizes are, you will have the capacity to eyeball portions and will have the capacity to get rid of calorie counting.

In the event that however your weight reduction begins to back off, you may need to execute it again just in the event that you are incidentally eating more than you ought to.

Chapter 7:

Some Mistakes to Avoid

Alright, so it's the ideal opportunity for the hard truth-for those of you waiting for the catch, here it is-changing over to a low-carb diet might be troublesome, in any event at first. Essentially, you are switching up the way that your body needs to get things done and making it work harder simultaneously. This won't go over so well at first and you can hope to feel just as you have influenza while the body is making this conformity.

The seriousness of the "withdrawal" side effects and span of this time of alteration will vary among one individual the other thus it is difficult to state what you will experience. The symptoms will undoubtedly be more awful for you in the event that you went from eating a diet high in refined carbs.

Luckily you will probably just need to bear the side effects for around three to seven days or somewhere close to that and there is a great chance that you can improve. For 90% of individuals, this diet is more in line the way that they ought to eat every day. For the remaining 10%, this diet is not going to work and can be harmful to your health if followed for an extended period.

Clearly you should be guided by your body and you have to utilize some judgment skills too. Try not to plan the first week of this diet for an especially occupied or distressing period for you. Here are approaches to guarantee that the change is as simple as possible & what to attempt if the diet does not appear to work for you.

Rule 1: Adhere to the guidelines entirely and change when and if fundamental to do so

Pay special attention to the signs that your body has gone into ketosis and alter the amounts of macronutrients as and where vital in case it is most certainly not. Sometimes even simply tweaking the proportions two or three

percentage points in either direction can be the distinction amongst success
& failure.

Rule 2: Work out the proportions and reassess as you get more fit

You will lose weight if at all you wing it however it is far much better to set
aside the time to really compute the ideal proportions. It is truly that
essential in the event that you are serious about rolling out a lasting
improvement in your life. It doesn't take that long at all: Work out the
quantity of aggregate calories vital for the day and afterward work out the
aggregate number of carbs, proteins and fats that you can eat regarding
ideal proportions.

Carbs: You may need to do some fine-tuning here in light of the fact that
everybody is unique. For some individuals going into ketosis implies
remaining at 5% total consumption of carbs. For others, this may just be
too low. Monitor your outcomes and see what works for you.

You should know about the distinction amongst aggregate and net carbs
here. To discover what the net carbs in a specific food are, take the
aggregate carb count & subtract the aggregate grams of fiber.

Fat: Fat is the other one to work out. Take your aggregate calorie count &
multiply it by 60-75%. Divide the resultant figure by 9 to get the quantity of
grams of fat that you can eat regularly.

Proteins: Whatever calorie count is left over, should originate from protein.
Improve the general calorie count by 15-20% & divide this aggregate by 4.
(1 gram of protein contains 4 calories).

Rule 3: Avoid banned foods

Before you begin, check your grocery cupboards and drawers and evacuate
any banned foods which may be present. It is ideal to get temptation out of
the way, particularly when you begin this plan. Make sure you avoid those
aisles in the store.

In case that is impossible for you, give yourself the most ideal possibility by planning your shopping tips carefully. Ensure that you have had a snack before going shopping-nothing blunts your judgment skills like feeling somewhat hungry & ensure that you make a list & just purchase what is on the list. Shop when you are not under pressure &, ideally, on the calmer days of the week, for instance Wednesday rather than Saturday-the grocery store will undoubtedly have all the more enticing newly baked goods throughout the end of the week than amid the week.

In the event that you are still not losing weight, or in the event that you are not feeling incredible on the plan after the initial modification stage, one of the following might be an issue:

Mistake 1: Eating Hidden Carbs

What precisely is a low-carb diet? There are many responses to this however as a rule, carb intake of between 100 grams to 150 grams every day is viewed as low and it is a considerable measure lower than what many people following a typical Western diet take in. In the event that you slice back to this level, you will undoubtedly lose some weight.

Just 5 percent of your calories are originating from sugars. There's no space for errors here! You have to eat a much of green verdant vegetables, nuts, and seeds, yet you likewise need to keep an eye out for the hidden sugars that are in processed foods.

Food organizations have moved toward becoming experts at concealing sugars in foods. They want you to be addicted to carbs. It's what drives their benefits! Along these lines, you should be your own best backer and turn into a specialist at reading food labels.

When you purchase something, perceive what number of carbs is listed in the sustenance facts; however similarly as essentially, look at the list of ingredients to check whether you can perceive any different names for sugars. A few are sucrose, fructose, rice syrup, lactose, dextrose, rice syrup, maltose, agave, molasses, cane juice, fruit juice, honey, and malt syrup.

These are the main ones; however they're unquestionably by all account not the only ones. In the event that you have any questions, don't buy it!

Mistake 2: Eating Too Much Protein

Protein is critical in our diets-we require it to help support sentiments of satiety and to rev up fat burning. However, the more protein you eat the more fat you will lose. In case you are eating more protein than your body can utilize, the amino acids in the abundance will be changed over into glucose. This thus, will keep you from achieving full ketosis

Various individuals can deal with various measures of protein once they're really fat-adjusted. However, in the early stages, it's ideal to be safe than sorry. What ends up happening in the event that you consume excessive protein on this diet is a procedure called gluconeogenesis. Basically, your body will treat that protein like sugars and change it over into glucose. That will remove you out of ketosis.

It's critical that you select high-fat, low-protein foods. You're not going to eat much chicken. You are not going to eat a lot of fish. When you go to the store, purchase the full-fat ground meat, not the ground turkey. Purchase the normal bacon rather than the turkey bacon. You just need 20 percent of your calories to originate from protein.

Mistake 3: Not Eating Enough Fat

The most ideal approach to consider keto is that it's not just a low-carb diet; it's a super-high-fat diet. Of course, you won't eat a ton of carbs, however it's fundamental that you change your outlook from one of "avoid carbs" to just "get enough fat."

Not less than 75 percent of your calories should originate from fat; that is things like eggs, bacon, wiener, avocado, oils, coconut oils, and margarine. You have to search these things out. Rationally, it's not what you're used to. You're accustomed to staying away from fats. Presently, all of a sudden, you take a gander at the grocery cart, and you have only fat.

That is something to be thankful for. Fat is your new energy source. You're not running on carbs any longer. You require fat. In the event that you don't get enough fat, your energy levels will go down, and you will end up stopping this diet.

In the event that you are on a ketogenic diet, you ought to never feel hungry. In case you are feeling hungry there is a chance that you are eating too minimal fat.

Mistake 4: Not Getting Enough Electrolytes

Electrolytes are vital regardless of how you eat, yet they're completely basic on this diet. Truth be told, they are the main motivation behind why many people end up losing weight. In the event that you don't have enough sodium, magnesium, and potassium in your diet, you will encounter headaches, exhaustion, constipation —as such, every one of the symptoms of the alleged "keto influenza"— and you will essentially stop.

Why does this happen? For one, insulin happens to be the hormone that advises your kidneys to store sodium. In this way, when you smother the insulin, your kidneys start flushing out the sodium from your body, particularly when you work out. It's basic that you supplant that sodium by salting your food, eating salty snacks, and drinking chicken broth.

Potassium is likewise a noteworthy electrolyte that is utilized as a part of every single diverse sort of muscle contractions and by your major organs. To get enough potassium, you can eat bunches of green verdant vegetables and avocados. Truly, it is advisable to eat 1-2 whole avocados a day. These little fat bombs can be your best companion!

At last, there's magnesium, which is utilized as a part of practically every chemical procedure in your body. You can get magnesium from nuts and seeds like walnuts, almonds, pistachios, pecans, and pumpkin seeds, all of which are on the menu with keto. In any case, it is likewise advisable to take some extra magnesium in supplemental form.

Mistake 5: Getting Impatient With Adaptation

Before you hop into keto, you need to comprehend something: You've been running on carbs your whole life. Presently you're asking your body to totally switch digestion systems and begin utilizing fat for energy rather than carbs.

You will have some withdrawal impacts amid this time, normally known as the "keto influenza." What you have to do is remain dedicated. There are approaches to limit the keto influenza, regardless of the possibility that you can't kill it totally. Continue up to the end, this season's flu virus will pass, and unexpectedly, you will be in ketosis, and you will feel superior to when you initially began.

Mistake 6: Comparing yourself to others

Stop. Simply stop. Another person's progress is not a determining component in your prosperity. Everybody is unique. We as a whole pick up and lose fat in various areas and at various rates. In case you get yourself continually basing your prosperity with respect to another person's progress, then you're treating it terribly. Because Skinny Sally lost 100 pounds in a month doesn't mean you are a failure in the event that you haven't. Because Thin Thomas slice his muscle to fat quotients to 10% doesn't mean you are a failure since you haven't. Everybody is unique. You need to realize what works for you. In any case, what doesn't work is attempting to contrast yourself and your success with other individuals. That is a formula for failure.

Mistake 7: You are going it alone

Rolling out an improvement in your life is possible, and it's exceptionally hard to support on the off chance that you aren't ready. You will be vastly improved off with a supportive group(it doesn't need to be an big group) of individuals who comprehend your struggle, comprehend your prosperity, and comprehend your adventure. Discover somebody who can be there to help, to caution, and to stroll with you.

Mistake 8: You are eating the wrong sorts of fat

It's insufficient to eat loads of fat. It must be the correct sorts of fats. To put it plainly, avoid vegetable and seed oils, the kind in the plastic holders. They are to a great degree unhealthy and will undermine every of your endeavors. You ought to eat soaked fats (animal fats, margarine, coconut oil), fish oil, and monounsaturated fat (olive oil).

Mistake 9: You are eating processed "keto" foods

Keto is about whole food, genuine food, real foods. You ought to eat ingredients. Try not to eat stuff that comes in individual wrappers. Quest bars, Atkins bars, and so forth are not real keto foods. They are setbacks & mishaps. They are candy bars wearing "affirmed" clothing. This isn't to imply that that you ought to never have one. Sometimes it may be all the best you can do, however the MAJORITY of your food ought to be genuine food, real food. You know… ingredients.

Mistake 10: You are not all in

Keto is not for the apathetic. You need to commit. It requires genuine assurance and grit. You're going against the grain & you're picking a lifestyle that is troublesome for the larger part of society to get it. You have to be decided. You completely should be all in. From a functional point of view, eating high fat and high carb (not conferring completely to keto) is a hazardous mix. You're picking the most noticeably awful conceivable situation and taking and risking your health. The appropriate response, obviously, is to commit completely to keto and receive the benefits of focused assurance and discipline.

Mistake 11: Focusing on the Scale

Ketogenic diets claim to individuals since they permit many individuals to rapidly lose a considerable measure of the weight. You most likely began it subsequent to hearing of somebody who lost 20 or 30 pounds in a brief timeframe. In case you don't get those same outcomes, you may be baffled.

However, the scale doesn't recount the entire story. You can thin down without seeing a lot of a distinction on the scale. Also, individuals who have more weight to lose have a tendency to lose that weight rapidly. In the event that you just need to lose 20 pounds to achieve your objective weight, it's most likely not going to all fall off in a month.

Rather, concentrate in the manner your body looks and feels. On the off chance that you have more energy and your clothes are feeling more comfortable, then you're seeing achievement, regardless of the possibility that it's not appearing on the scale.

Mistake 12: You're stressed

Another oversight on keto individuals make is not resting enough and being excessively worried. It can likewise be the mystery thing that prevents you from getting into ketosis in any case.

In case there are excessively numerous stress factors throughout your life, you'll discharge more adrenaline and glucose into your circulatory system. This frustrates the usage of ketone bodies and puts an end to the adaptation procedure.

Each time you get furious or shout at somebody in activity, you're raising your blood glucose levels and turn into a seething sugar burner. Nobody needs to associate with somebody like that.

Mistake 13: Keto sticks

Individuals utilize sticks believing that it is disclosing to them what state of their body is in, in case they are in ketosis or not. Exceptionally improbable, it is not precise. The issue with keto sticks is that you drink a lot of water; you will have a diluted reading. It doesn't mean how many- it is not disclosing to you how much ketones are in your blood, it's the abundant ketones coming out, which is another element. We would prefer not to read what is leaving your body. It is in all likelihood since you have high glucose and high ketones, which are an awful domain, yet your body, will utilize keto-the glucose and after that simply remove the ketones, so you are reading the wrong thing.

Mistake 14: Drinking alcohol routinely

Some alcoholic drinks are low in carbs, so in fact, you can have them. However, liquor can influence your weight reduction in other impeding ways. It converts to empty calories. It meddles with absorption of different supplements, as your body will dependably process liquor first. Liquor can likewise disturb your hormonal balance & make weight reduction harder. You may believe that one little glass of wine each other day can't do any damage. However, as a general rule, this could be the variable bringing about your weight reduction blunder. Try to remove it totally.

Conforming to the Ketogenic diet and way of life is a process, and, similar to whatever other procedure, there are some hindrances. These bends and bumps can prompt dissatisfaction, however they don't need to. So, those are the most well-known mistakes people are doing on keto. Some of them are mental, some are functional, and some are passionate. Low-carb diet is an incredible approach to lose weight. Keep an eye out for these basic mistakes and get the full advantages of this way of life.

Chapter 8:

Breakfast recipes

Many healthy eaters struggle with breakfast. Some are busy in the morning; others simply don't feel hungry at the start of the day. Many people also feel so satiated on a low-carb diet that the need for a morning meal vanishes. If this applies to you, then perhaps you should just skip breakfast and wait until you naturally want to eat.

But for those who feel and perform better with breakfast, it is crucial to start your day with something protein rich and healthy. Having a processed cereal is the absolute worst thing you can eat at the start of the day. Below we have listed some ideas for delicious keto breakfasts. We hope you'll like them and that they will help you achieve your health goals.

a)   Fake Meat-Based Pizza... Meatza

If you miss pizza, then you're going to love this. It tastes even better, in our opinion, without all the nasty ingredients. This recipe is very easy to modify and you can add whatever you want to it be it vegetables, mushrooms, different cheeses, etc.

Ingredients:

- Ground Beef
- Salsa
- Onions
- Spice
- Garlic Powder
- Shredded Cheese
- Bacon

Instructions:

1. Cut onions into little pieces and bacon into small slices.

2. Mix ground beef, salsa, onions, spices and garlic powder at the bottom of a baking dish.

3. Add shredded cheese on top.

4. Spread bacon slices over the whole thing.

5. Insert into oven, heat at 180-200°C (356-392°F) for 30-40 minutes, until bacon and cheese look crunchy.

b) Cheeseburgers without the Bun

This is a meal worth trying. Burgers without the bun, with some cheeses and served with raw spinach.

Ingredients:

- Butter
- Hamburgers
- Cheddar Cheese
- Cream Cheese
- Salsa
- Spices
- Spinach

Instructions:

1. Put butter on pan, turn up the heat.

2. Add burgers and spices.

3. Flip until close to being ready.

4. Add a few slices of cheddar and some cream cheese on top.

5. Turn down the heat and put a lid on the pan until the cheese melts.

6.   Serve with some spinach. I like to pour some of the fat from the pan on top of the spinach.

7.   To make the burgers even juicier, add some salsa on top.

c) Ground Beef with Sliced Bell Peppers

This is a meal you should eat from time to time, not very often. It is perfect if you have some spare ground beef lying around.

Ingredients:

- Coconut Oil
- Onions
- Ground Beef
- Spinach
- Spices
- Bell Pepper

Instructions:

1.   Cut an onion in little pieces.

2.   Put coconut oil on pan, turn up the heat.

3.   Add onion to pan, stir for a minute or two.

4.   Add ground beef.

5.   Add some spices (I use a spice mix, but salt and pepper work fine).

6.   Add spinach.

7.   (Optional) if you want to spice things up a bit, add some black pepper and chili powder.

d) Bacon and Eggs

Bacon wouldn't exactly be called a health food. It is processed meat, after all. But it is still low in carbs and you can eat it on a low-carb diet and still lose weight. I personally eat bacon and eggs once or twice a week.

Ingredients:

- Bacon
- Eggs

Instructions:

1. Add bacon to pan, fry until ready.
2. Put the bacon on a plate; fry a few eggs (I use 3-4) in the bacon fat.
3. (Optional) If you want to add some flavor to the eggs, put a bit of sea salt, garlic powder and onion powder on them while frying.

e) Grilled Chicken Wings with Greens and Salsa

This is one of all-time favorite meals. There's something "primitive" about eating meat off the bone.

Ingredients:

- Chicken Wings
- Spices
- Some Greens
- Salsa

Instructions:

1. Put spice on chicken wings (I use a chicken spice mix).

2.   Insert into oven, heat at 180-200°C (356-392°F) for about 40 minutes.

3.   Grill until wings are brown and crunchy.

4.   Serve with some vegetables and salsa.

f) Eggs and Vegetables, Fried in Coconut Oil

This is what you should eat for breakfast literally every single day. I never get tired of it and it keeps me full for a long time.

Ingredients:

- Coconut oil
- Spinach
- Frozen Vegetable Mix (carrots, cauliflower, broccoli, green beans)
- Spices

Instructions:

1.   Add coconut oil to frying pan and turn up the heat.

2.   Add vegetables. 3. Add eggs (use 3 or 4).

3.   Add spices. Use a spice mix, although salt and pepper work great too.

4.   (Optional) Add spinach.

5.   Stir fry until ready.

g) Mushroom Omelet

Ingredients:

- 3 eggs
- 7/8 oz. butter, for frying

- 7/8 oz. shredded cheese
- 1/5 yellow onion
- 2 – 3 mushrooms
- salt and pepper

Instructions

1. Crack the eggs into a mixing bowl with a pinch of salt and pepper. Whisk the eggs into a batter with a fork.
2. Add salt and spices.
3. Melt butter in a frying pan and pour in the batter when the butter has melted.
4. When the omelet begins to cook and get firm, but still has a little raw egg on top, sprinkle cheese, mushrooms and onion on top (optional).
5. Using a spatula, ease around the edges of the omelet, and then fold it over in half. When it starts to turn golden brown underneath, remove the pan from the heat and slide the omelet on to a plate.

h) Keto Breakfast Banana Chia Pudding

Ingredients:

- 1 can coconut milk (full fat)
- 1 medium or small size banana, ripe
- ½ teaspoon cinnamon
- ½ teaspoon salt
- 1 teaspoon vanilla extract
- ¼ cup chia seeds

Instructions:

1. In a medium size bowl mash the banana until soft.

2. Combine the rest of the ingredients and mix until combined

3. Cover and place in the refrigerator overnight.

4. Enjoy when ready

i)   Cheesy Buffalo Scrambled Mug Eggs

Ingredients:

*   Coffee mug

*   2 eggs

*   Salt and pepper

*   Your favorite buffalo wing sauce

Instructions:

1. Crack eggs into a coffee mug, whisk eggs with fork

2. Put the mug into your microwave and cook for 1.5-2 minutes, depending on the power of your microwave

3. Remove the mug from the microwave

4. Sprinkle with salt and pepper

5. Add on your desired amount of cheese

6. Using a folk, mix everything together

7. Add your favorite buffalo or sauce and mix again

8. Serve and enjoy

j)   Keto Egg, cheese and bacon biscuits

Ingredients:

*   1 cup almond flour

- 4 egg whites
- 1/3 cup grass-fed butter
- 1t baking powder
- ½ t salt
- 4 pieces of speck, prosciutto, pancetta, bacon or sausage patties, cooked crispy
- 4 eggs, fried
- 4 slices raw, grass-fed sharp cheddar cheese
- 4 tablespoon of your favorite jam

Instructions:

Biscuits

1. In a mixer add together butter and almond flour and mix until you have small broken up bits of butter.
2. Add the eggs whites, salt, and baking powder and mix well.
3. On a greased or lined baking sheet scoop the butter into 4 even portions.
4. Bake at 350F about 20 minutes, until slightly golden.

To Assemble

1. Cut the biscuits in half, spread jam on top or bottom.
2. Put the egg, then the cheese followed by whichever meat you have crisped up.
3. Place the other half of the biscuit on top and enjoy.

k) Kristy's Ketogen pancakes

Ingredients:

- 1 scoop of KetogenX Vanilla
- 1 tablespoon of almond or hazelnut meal
- 2 tablespoons water
- 1 egg

Instructions:

1. Add together ingredients in a bowl
2. In a non-stick pan cook on moderate heat for approximately 2 t0 3 minutes on each side
3. Watch carefully as it may burn quickly
4. Serve buttered with a handful of mixed berries

l) Keto egg porridge

Ingredients:

- 2 organic free-range eggs
- 1/3 cup organic heavy cream without food additives
- 2 packages NuStieva or your preferred sweetener to taste
- 2 tablespoons grass-fed butter
- Ground organic cinnamon to taste

Instructions:

1. In a small bowl add together eggs, cream and the sweetener and whisk together
2. Melt the butter in a medium sauce pan over medium high-heat. Lower the heat to the minimum once the butter is melted
3. Combine the egg and cream mixture
4. Cook, all the time mixing along the bottom until the mixture thickens and starts curdling.

5. When you see the first signs of curdling, remove the saucepan immediately from heat.

6. Pour the porridge in a serving bowl. Sprinkle plenty of cinnamon on top and serve immediately.

m) Cheesy pancakes

Ingredients:

- 2 oz. full fat cream cheese
- 2 large eggs
- 1 tablespoon coconut flour
- ½ teaspoon powdered cinnamon
- ½ sachet stevia powder

Instructions:

1. Beat together everything well and fry in coconut oil or ghee over a medium heat until done, in the same way as you would any other pancakes flipping once.

2. Serve piping hot!

n) Granola Keto Style

Ingredients:

- 5 tablespoons flaked coconut
- 7 tablespoons ground hemp seeds
- 5 tablespoons ground flaxseed
- 2 tablespoons psyllium husk
- 2 tablespoons ground sesame seeds
- 2 tablespoons dark cocoa powder(no added sugar)

Instructions:

1.   Mix together everything and refrigerate until ready to eat.

2.   Serve with full fat cream or with little water.

o) Low carb bread

Ingredients:

- 1 ½ cup finely ground almond flour
- 3 large eggs, whites only- reserve yolks for another dish
- ½ cup full fat Coconut milk ½ cup pureed pumpkin
- ¼ psyllium powder
- ¼ cup powdered swerve
- 1 ½ teaspoon pumpkin pie spice
- 2 teaspoons baking powder
- ½ teaspoon salt

Instructions:

1.   Warm up your oven to a temperature of 350F. separate the dry and wet ingredients and combine

2.   Set a ramekin filled with water on the lowest oven rack

3.   Mix the milk and puree together and fold into the dry ingredients.

4.   Whisk the egg whites till soft peak stage has been reached and then fold them in as well

5.   Mix dough is smooth

6.   Spray a loaf tin with baking spray and put the dough in it

7.   Bake for about an hour and a quarter

p) Keto eggs Florentine

Ingredients:

- 1 cup washed, fresh spinach leaves
- 2 tablespoons freshly grated parmesan cheese
- Sea salt and pepper to taste
- 1 tablespoon white vinegar
- 2 eggs

Instructions

1. Cook spinach in a microwave safe bowl in microwave or steam until wilted
2. Sprinkle with parmesan cheese and season to taste
3. Slice into bite size pieces and place on a plate
4. Heat a pan of simmering water, adding the vinegar and stir with wooden spoon to create a whirl pool
5. Break an egg into the center, turn off the heat and leave covered until set (3-4 minutes).
6. Repeat with second egg.
7. Place eggs on spinach and serve.

q) Lorraine

Ingredients:

Crust

- 1 ½ cups blanched almond flour
- 1 ½ freshly grated parmesan cheese
- ¼ teaspoon Celtic sea salt
- 1 egg

Swiss sauce

- 1 tablespoon butter
- ½ cup chicken/beef broth
- 1 cup grated Swiss cheese
- 4 ounce cream cheese
- 1 teaspoon Celtic sea salt

Filling

- 12 slices bacon
- Cheese sauce
- 1/3 cup minced leeks
- 4 eggs, beaten
- ¾ teaspoon sea salt
- 1/8 teaspoon cayenne pepper

Instructions:

1. Preheat the oven to 325 degrees F
2. For the tart shell
3. Add together the flour, cheese and salt and mix well
4. Combine the egg and mix until the dough is well combined and stiff
5. Press pie crust into pie dish or tart pan
6. Bake the crust for 12-15 minutes, or until it starts to lightly brown

To make cheese sauce

1. Melt the butter in a medium saucepan over medium heat

2. Add in the rest of the ingredients and mix; season with the salt and pepper

3. Meanwhile, place bacon in a large skillet and fry over medium-high heat until crisp

4. Drain on paper towels, then slice coarsely

5. Spread bacon into pastry shell

6. In a medium bowl, whisk together cheese, sauce, leeks, eggs, salt and cayenne pepper

7. Pour the mixture into pastry shell

8. Bake 15 minutes in the preheated oven

9. Reduce heat to 300 degrees F and bake an additional 30 minutes or until a knife inserted 1 inch from edge comes out

10. Let cool and enjoy

Chapter 9:

Main meal recipes

a)   **Chicken in Herb Cream Sauce**

Ingredients:

- 5 tablespoons butter, divided
- 2 small white onions, thinly sliced
- 3 large garlic cloves
- ½ cup chicken broth
- ½ cup dry white wine
- 8 oz. cream cheese
- ½ cup heavy cream
- 1 tsp. dried tarragon
- 1 ½ tsp. Herbes De Provence
- 1 tsp. Weber Canadian Chicken Seasoning
- Salt to taste
- 4 raw chicken breasts

Instructions:

1. Over medium heat, sauté onions, garlic and tarragon in 2 tablespoons of butter until soft. Remove from skillet and set aside.

2. In same skillet, add 2 tablespoons of butter and melt over low heat. Add wine. Add cream cheese and stir until melted and mixed with the wine and butter. Add cream and spices and stir until mixed.

3.   Preheat oven to 350 degrees F. Use 1 tablespoon of butter to grease a 9/13 glass baking dish. Pour chicken broth into baking dish.

4.   Add chicken to baking dish in a single layer.

5.   Spoon the onion mixture over the chicken in even proportions.

6.   Spoon the cream sauce mixture over chicken and onions. Bake at 350 degrees for 45 minutes to one hour.

7.   Serve with a salad. Makes 4 servings.

b) Chicken Guadalajara

Ingredients:

- 2-3 tablespoons butter
- 4 ounces of white onion, chopped fine
- 3 garlic cloves, minced
- 4 boneless, skinless, chicken breast halves
- 2- 6oz cans diced tomatoes and green chilies
- 4 oz. full fat cream cheese, cut into slices or cubes
- ¼ cup whipping cream
- ¼ cup chicken broth
- ½ teaspoon cayenne pepper (to taste)
- 1 teaspoon dried cumin
- ½ teaspoon garlic powder to taste
- 1 teaspoon sea salt
- grated cheddar cheese for garnish
- sour cream for garnish
- salsa for garnish

Instructions:

1. Wash and pat dry chicken breasts, slice across in ½" slices.

2. In a medium skillet, over medium heat, melt butter and sauté onions and garlic until soft.

3. Add chicken, and using spatula turn to cook all sides of slices until juices run clear.

4. Decrease heat to medium low, and add tomatoes, spices and chilies. Cover, and allow chicken to simmer for another 8-10 minutes.

5. Add cream cheese and cream, and stir until cheese is melted, and chicken and vegetables are coated. Add broth to thin if sauce is too thick.

6. Makes 4 servings. Top with garnishes if desired.

c) Herb Baked Salmon

The herbs used in this recipe are dried. If you're using fresh, you may want to increase the amounts a bit since dried herbs are much stronger.

Ingredients:

- 2 pounds salmon fillets
- 4 ounces sesame oil
- 1/2 cup tamari soy sauce
- 1 teaspoon minced garlic
- 1/2 teaspoon ground ginger
- 1/2 teaspoon basil
- 1 teaspoon oregano leaves
- 1/4 teaspoon thyme
- 1/2 teaspoon rosemary

- 1/4 teaspoon tarragon
- 4 ounces butter
- 1/2 cup chopped fresh mushrooms
- 1/2 cup chopped green onions

Instructions:

1. If you have one large, single fillet cut it into 1/2 pound pieces. Get a quart size freezer style Ziploc bag.
2. Stir together the tamari sauce, sesame oil and spices. Put the salmon into the Ziploc bag and pour in the sauce mixture.
3. Refrigerate the salmon, skin side up, in the marinade for 1-4 hours.
4. Preheat oven to 350 degrees F. Line a large baking pan with foil.
5. Pour out the fillets and marinade into the pan. The fish should be in a single layer.
6. Bake fillets for 10-15 minutes.
7. While the salmon is baking, get vegetables ready.
8. Melt the butter. Add the vegetables to it, and mix to coat vegetables.
9. Remove the salmon from the oven, and pour the butter mixture over the salmon fillets, making sure each fillet gets covered.
10. Bake at 350 degrees F. for about 10 minutes more. Serve immediately.

d) Roasted Brussels sprouts and Prosciutto Bites

Ingredients:

- 1 pound small Brussels sprouts, rinsed of any dirt
- 2 tablespoons extra-virgin olive oil
- ¼ pound thinly sliced prosciutto
- 1 pinch coarse salt and freshly ground pepper

Instructions:

1. Preheat the oven to 400 degrees F
2. Slice the Brussels sprouts into halves, lengthwise (do not burn trim the ends as they will hold together better with them)
3. Toss the sprouts on a rimmed baking sheet with oil and sprinkle with salt and pepper.
4. Bake for up 40 minutes, but begin checking at around the 25 minute mark. Feel free to toss them around a bit too.
5. Chop the prosciutto into small chunks.
6. Heat a medium-sized skillet over medium to high heat.
7. Add the prosciutto and sauté for about 5 minutes, or until you can handle them.
8. Use a toothpick to slide on a couple of sprout halves, followed by a slice or 3 of the ham, then bookend it with another sprout half.
9. Continue this way until you have about 32 mini skewers.
10. Arrange on a platter and serve immediately.

e) Easy Keto skirt steak fajitas

Ingredients:

- 1 small onion
- 1 medium bell pepper
- 3 medium jalapenos

- 1 small red chili pepper

- 2 lbs. skirt steak

- 2 teaspoon cumin

- ½ can whole tomatoes

- 1 tablespoon apple cider vinegar

- 3 tablespoon ketchup

- 1 tablespoon liquid smoke

- 1 teaspoon minced garlic

- Salt & pepper

Tortillas

- ¼ cup coconut flour

- 1 tablespoon ground psyllium husk

- 2 tablespoon butter

- ½ cup chicken or beef broth

- 1 pinch garlic powder

- 1 pinch seasoning salt

Instructions:

1. Remove silver skin from skirt steak if your butcher missed any

2. Cut up all vegetables into bite-size pieces

3. Remove seeds from jalapenos and red chili if you don't like much spice

4. Combine all ingredients

5. Cook on low for 6-8 hours

6. When you are ready make your tortillas by boiling the broth and then mixing it into the other ingredients

7. Form a dough and cut small circles out

8. Fry each circle in a pan on the stove until they have browned. Add fillings of your choice.

9. Enjoy!

f) Keto chicken satay

Ingredients:

- 1 lb. ground chicken
- 4 tablespoon soy sauce
- 3 tablespoon peanut butter
- 2 spring onions
- 1/3 yellow pepper
- 1 tablespoon Erythritol
- 1 tablespoon rice vinegar
- 2 teaspoon sesame oil
- 2 teaspoon chili paste
- 1 teaspoon minced garlic
- ¼ teaspoon cayenne
- ¼ teaspoon paprika
- Juice of ½ lime

Instructions:

1. Heat 2 teaspoons sesame oil on medium-high heat in a pan
2. Add chicken to the pan and cook until brown
3. Once chicken is cooked, add all other ingredients
4. Stir well and continue cooking
5. Once everything is cooked, add 2 chopped spring onions and 1/3 sliced yellow pepper for garnish

g) Keto cauliflower and curry shrimp

Ingredients:

- 24 oz. shrimp
- 5 cups raw spinach
- 4 cups chicken stock
- 1 medium onion
- 1 teaspoon onion powder
- 1 teaspoon cayenne
- 1 teaspoon paprika
- ½ teaspoon ginger (ground, dried)
- ½ teaspoon coriander
- ½ teaspoon turmeric
- ½ teaspoon pepper
- ¼ teaspoon cardamom
- ¼ teaspoon cinnamon
- ¼ teaspoon xanthan gum
- Salt + pepper to taste
- ½ head medium cauliflower
- 1 cup unsweetened coconut milk
- ¼ cup butter
- ¼ cup heavy cream
- 3 tablespoon olive oil
- 2 tablespoon curry powder
- 1 tablespoon coconut floor
- 1 tablespoon cumin
- 2 teaspoon garlic powder
- 1 teaspoon chili powder

Instructions:

1. Stir all spices together (except xanthan and coconut flour) set aside.

2. Slice I medium onion into slices

3. Bring 3 tablespoon olive oil to hot heat in a pan. Add onion, cook onion till soft.

4. Add butter, heavy cream 1/8 teaspoon xanthan and spices sweating; add 4 cups chicken broth, and 1 cup coconut milk.

5. Mix well, cover and cook for thirty minutes.

6. Meanwhile, chop cauliflower into small florets then add to curry.

7. Cook for another 15 minutes, covered.

8. Add shrimp to the curry. Cook for an additional 10-20 minutes with the lid off.

9. Enjoy!

h) Keto turkey meatballs

Ingredients:

- 10 slices bacon
- 2 lbs. ground turkey
- 3 small red chilis
- ½ medium green pepper
- 1 small onion
- ½ teaspoon salt
- ½ teaspoon pepper
- 2 large handful spinach
- 3 springs thyme

- 2 large eggs
- 1 oz. pork rinds

Instructions:

1. Preheat the oven to 400F
2. Line a baking sheet with foil and add your bacon.
3. Cook for 30 minutes or until crisp.
4. Meanwhile, prep all ingredients by adding to food processor and dicing.
5. Add all ingredients (except bacon) to the ground turkey and mix well.
6. Once bacon is cooked, set bacon aside and drain fat into separate container.
7. Make 20 meatballs and lay over the same sheet the bacon cooked on.
8. Cook meatballs for 15-20 minutes or until juices run clear, and then skewer 2-3 pieces of bacon to each meatball.
9. In the food processor, combine spinach, bacon, fat, and seasonings of your choosing, create "stick" of butter and serve under meatballs.
10. Enjoy!

i) Keto roasted rosemary chicken thighs

Ingredients:

- 7 skinless, boneless chicken thigh
- 1 tablespoon minced garlic
- 3 tablespoon olive oil
- 2 large lemons

- 2 tablespoon fresh thyme
- 3 teaspoon kosher salt
- 1 ½ teaspoon dried Rosemary
- 1 ½ teaspoon dried ground sage
- ½ teaspoon ground black pepper

Instructions:

1. In a mortar, add garlic and 2 teaspoons kosher salt.
2. Grind the garlic and salt together with a pestle, creating a paste.
3. Slowly add your oil, grinding and mixing into a paste.
4. Once the paste is ready, dry your chicken off and put it into a bag with the paste.
5. Coat the chicken well.
6. Marinate the chicken for anywhere from 2-10 hours.
7. Preheat your oven to 425F.
8. Slice 2 lemons thin and arrange the slices on the bottom of baking pan.
9. Lay your chicken on top of the lemons.
10. Remove the thyme leaves from the stem and your thyme, rosemary, sage, pepper, and remaining salt to the chicken.
11. Bake for 25-30 minutes, or until the juices run clear.

j) Joseph's keto pita pizza

Ingredients:

- 1 joseph's low carb pita
- ½ cup Rao's homemade tomato basil marinara sauce
- 2 oz. cheddar cheese
- 1 oz. roasted red peppers

- 14slices pepperoni

Instructions:

1. Place half of the low carb pita on a foil lined sheet

2. Rub with some olive oil and crisp it by toasting for 1-2 minutes at 450F.

3. Spread the sauce over the pita bread then cover with cheese and toppings.

4. Cook for another five minutes to melt the cheese, then serve while hot.

k) Keto broccoli cheese pie

Ingredients:

- 1 average broccoli (8.8 oz.)

- 1 cup grated parmesan cheese (2.1 oz.)

- 3 large eggs (free range or organic)

- 4 tbsp. fresh full-fat cream

- 6 anchovies

- 2 tbsp. extra virgin olive oil

- Salt and pepper to taste

- ½ cup micro greens for garnish

Instructions:

1. Preheat the oven to 300F.

2. Cut the washed broccoli into florets

3. Transfer them into a steamer for about 5-8 minutes or until the stalks are slightly tender.

4. When done, transfer them into a bowl and blend until smooth.

5.   Add grated parmesan cheese, eggs and cream then mix well as you season with salt and pepper.

6.   Spoon the mixture into silicone forms equally (it is advisable to bake them in a water bath as this prevents the top part from drying and cracking)

7.   Place the silicone forms on a baking tray and add 2 cm or 1 inch of water into the tray.

8.   Place in the oven and bake it for 40 minutes, when this is done, set aside and let them cool.

9.   Finely chop the anchovies and mix them with olive oil.

10.   Remove the cakes from the forms once they are chilled, spoon anchovies on the top garnish with micro greens. Enjoy your meal now.

Chapter 10:

Dessert recipes

a)   Oven-Baked Brie Cheese

Ingredients:

- 8¾ oz. Brie cheese or Camembert cheese
- 2 oz. pecan nuts or walnuts
- 1 garlic clove
- 1 tablespoon fresh rosemary or fresh thyme or fresh parsley
- 1 tablespoon olive oil
- salt and pepper

Instructions:

1.   Preheat the oven to 400°F (200°C). Place the cheese on a sheet pan lined with parchment paper or in a small nonstick baking dish.

2.   Mince garlic and chop the nuts and herbs coarsely. Mix all three together with the olive oil. Add salt and pepper.

3.   Place the nut mixture on the cheese and bake for 10 minutes or until cheese is warm and soft and nuts are toasted. Serve warm or lukewarm.

b) Low-Carb Crustless Pumpkin Pie

Ingredients

- 2 tablespoons butter, for greasing the baking dish
- 4 tablespoons unsweetened shredded coconut
- 1 lb. pumpkins
- 2/3 cup heavy whipping cream
- 1 oz. butter
- ¼ teaspoon salt
- 2 teaspoons pumpkin pie spice
- 2 tablespoons rosehip flour (optional)
- ¼ lemon, only the zest
- 1 teaspoon baking powder
- 3 eggs
- 1½ cups heavy whipping cream, for serving

Instructions:

1. Dice the pumpkin into cubes and place in a pan. Pour cream, salt and butter on top. Bring to a boil.

2. Lower the heat, let simmer until the pumpkin is soft. It will take at least 15–20 minutes. Stir occasionally.

3. When the pumpkin is soft, add the rest of the ingredients, except for the eggs, and mix to a smooth puré using a hand mixer, blender or food processor.

4. Whisk the eggs in a separate bowl with a hand mixer for 2–3 minutes. Add the pumpkin puré and mix well.

5. Preheat the oven to 400°F (200°C). Grease a baking dish with butter and apply the coconut flakes evenly.

6.   Pour the batter into the baking dish and bake for 20 minutes.

7.   Serve with a dollop of whipped heavy cream.

c) Coconut Pancakes:

Ingredients:

- 6 eggs
- ½ cup coconut flour
- ¾ cup coconut milk
- 2 tablespoons melted coconut oil
- 1 pinch salt
- 1 teaspoon baking powder
- butter or coconut oil for frying

Instructions:

1.   Separate the yolk from the egg whites and whisk the egg whites vigorously with salt, preferably use a hand mixer. Continue whisking until stiff peaks form and then set aside.

2.   Whisk together yolks, oil and coconut milk in a different bowl.

3.   Add coconut flour and baking powder and mix into a smooth batter.

4.   Carefully fold the egg whites into the batter. Let sit for 5 minutes.

5.   Fry in butter or coconut oil for a couple of minutes or so on each side on low to medium heat.

6.   Serve with melted butter or fresh berries.

d) Keto Lemon Custard Tarts with Almond Lavender Crust

Ingredients:

For the crust

- 3 tbsp. unsalted butter, melted
- 3/4 cup almond meal
- 1/2 tbsp. dried lavender flowers (optional)
- 1 tbsp. sugar-free vanilla syrup (like Torani)

For the filling

- 4 large egg yolks
- grated zest of 3 lemons
- 1/2 cup unsalted butter, melted
- 1/2 cup freshly squeezed lemon juice
- 1/4-1/2 cup sugar-free vanilla syrup (depends on your preference for a zing, for instance you can use 1/4)

Instructions:

1. Preheat oven to 375 F
2. Take two creme brulee dishes (4.5 inches in diameter x 1.25 inches thick) and grease them (you can use ghee)
3. In a mortar and pestle, grind lavender flowers into a fine dust.
4. Mix lavender, almond flour, and 3 tbsp. melted butter
5. Press mix into the bottom of the dishes.
6. Bake for 10 minutes or until the tops begin to brown, then remove from oven and set aside.
7. In a blender or food processor, blend the egg yolks, lemon zest, lemon juice, sweetener, and 1/2 cup melted butter until smooth.

8.   Transfer filling to a small saucepan and cook over medium-low heat, stirring constantly with a spatula until thick like pudding (about 15 minutes).

9.   Pour the filling over the almond-lavender crust in the two dishes.

10.   Cover with plastic wrap and refrigerate overnight.

11.   Enjoy!

e) Sugar-Free Lavender Vanilla Syrup

Ingredients:

- 1 cup water
- 1 tablespoon organic culinary lavender
- ½ cup Erythritol
- 1 drop liquid stevia
- 1 teaspoon vanilla extract

Instructions:

1.   In a small saucepan, bring the water to a boil over high heat.

2.   Reduce the heat to low and mix in the lavender, Erythritol, stevia, and vanilla. Simmer for 5 minutes.

3.   Strain the syrup into a glass jar through several layers of cheesecloth or a fine-mesh strainer.

4.   Cover the jar and refrigerate for up to 2 weeks.

f) Buttery Chocolate Keto Fudge Squares

Ingredients:

- 3oz Baker's unsweetened chocolate squares

- 2 tbsp. ghee
- 1 tbsp. coconut oil
- 2 tbsp. butter
- 1/3 cup organic peanut butter (with no added sugars)
- 1 tbsp. sugar free vanilla syrup
- 1/3 cup sugar free maple syrup

Instructions:

1. Melt all of the above in a double broiler
2. Add to an 4x8 pan, lined with parchment paper
3. Freeze
4. Cut into pieces, and store in the refrigerator

g) Watermelon Cream Soup

Ingredients:

- ¾ cup seeded watermelon chunks
- ¼ cup raspberries
- 2 tablespoons organic sour cream
- 1 tablespoon Sugar-Free Vanilla Bean Sweetener
- ¼ teaspoon freshly squeezed lemon juice
- ¼ teaspoon chopped fresh mint
- 1/2 cup freshly whipped cream (made from whipping heavy cream)

Instructions:

1. In a blender, combine the watermelon, raspberries, sour cream, sweetener, lemon juice, and mint.

2.   Pulse until smooth.

3.   Pour the soup into a small bowl and top with the whipped cream. Serve immediately.

h) Low Carb Cheesecake Filled Strawberries

Ingredients:

- 10 small strawberries (or 5 large ones)
- 3 oz. cream cheese
- 1 tbsp. sugar-free vanilla syrup
- 1/4 cup almond flour

Instructions:

1.   Pour the almond flour onto a plate and spread out.

2.   Heat the cream cheese in the microwave for 15 seconds.

3.   Add the sugar-free vanilla syrup and mix.

4.   Use a spoon or pipette to add the cream cheese mixture into the strawberries.

5.   Press the top of your strawberry into the plate of almond flour.

6.   Do this to all your strawberries, then refrigerate for 30 minutes and enjoy!

i) Keto Unbaked Strawberry Muffin

Ingredients:

- 1 oz. cream cheese
- 1 tbsp. unsalted butter
- 1 tbsp. Steviva Blend + 1 tbsp. hot water, mixed (or 2 tbsps. sugar-free vanilla syrup)

- 1/2 tsp. vanilla extract

- 1 tbsp. coconut flour

- 2 tbsps. almond flour

- 3 strawberries (chopped)

Instructions:

1. In a mug, melt cream cheese and butter in the microwave (or in a saucepan if you prefer).

2. Add Steviva Blend, hot water, and vanilla extracts and mix.

3. Add the coconut flour and almond flour and mix again.

4. Finally, add in chopped strawberries and mix into a dough, then enjoy!

j) Low Carb Blackberry Chocolate Chip Cake

Ingredients:

- 2 cups almond flour

- 1 cup unsweetened shredded coconut

- 1/2 Swerve Sweetener / Erythritol

- 1/4 cup chocolate whey protein powder

- 2 tsp. baking soda

- 1/4 tsp. salt

- 4 large eggs

- 1/4 cup coconut oil (melted)

- 1/4 cup ghee (melted)

- 1/2 cup heavy cream

- 1 cup blackberries (washed)

- 1/3 cup dark / sugar free chocolate chips

Optional Topping

- 1 cup blackberries
- 1 sage leaf

Instructions:

1. Grease the inside of a standard 6 quart slow cooker with ghee. I used Tin Star Foods brown butter ghee because it's OMG so good.

2. Mix together the almond flour, coconut, sweetener, whey protein powder, baking soda and salt.

3. Stir in eggs, melted coconut oil, ghee, and heavy cream until well combined. Gently fold in blackberries and chocolate chips, if using.

4. Spread batter in prepared slow cooker and cook on low for 3 hours. Turn off slow cooker and let cake cool completely.

5. As an optional topping (highly recommended), in the microwave, add the second cup of blackberries and heat for 30 seconds, covered. Add sage leaf and blend.

6. When cake cools, use a spatula to gently remove the cake, and top with blackberry compote.

7. You can also heat up later and add butter!

k) Berry-Sage Fruit Salad in a Vanilla Bean Mascarpone Dressing (Low Carb)

Ingredients:

- 1 cup of mixed berries (strawberries, raspberries, blueberries, blackberries)
- 1 sage leaf, chopped

- 2 tbsp. mascarpone
- 1/2 vanilla bean (scoop out the inside)
- 1/2 tbsp. heavy cream

Instructions:

1. In one bowl mix berries and chopped sage.
2. In another bowl, mix together mascarpone cheese, vanilla bean pulp and heavy cream.
3. Microwave cream mixture for 10 seconds and mix.
4. Add cream to mixed berries and enjoy.

I) Low-Carb Chocolate Mousse

Ingredients:

- 3 1/3 cups coconut milk
- 2 – 3 tablespoons cocoa powder
- 1 teaspoon vanilla extract
- 1 teaspoon honey (optional)

Instructions:

1. Let the coconut milk sit in the fridge for 4 hours or longer to separate the cream from the coconut water.
2. Open the can carefully and scoop out the thick cream with a spoon and put in a bowl. Save the coconut water for a smoothie or pancakes.
3. Whisk the coconut cream, vanilla and optional honey with a hand mixer for a couple of minutes until it thickens. Add cocoa powder and whisk some more.
4. Serve in dessert bowls.

m) Frozen Yogurt Popsicles

Ingredients:

- ½ lb. frozen mango, diced
- ½ lb. frozen strawberries
- 1 cup Greek yogurt
- 8 tablespoons heavy whipping cream
- 1 teaspoon vanilla extract

Instructions:

1. Let mango and strawberries thaw for 10–15 minutes.
2. Put all the ingredients in a blender and mix until smooth.
3. Serve immediately as soft serve ice cream or pour into popsicle forms and let freeze for at least a couple of hours. If you have an ice cream maker you can of course use that.

n) Low-Carb Chocolate and Hazelnut Spread

Ingredients:

- 1/3 lb. hazelnuts
- 31/3 tablespoons coconut oil
- 1 oz. butter
- 1 – 2 tablespoons cocoa powder
- 1 teaspoon vanilla extract

Instructions:

1. Roast the hazelnuts in a dry and hot frying pan until they turn a nice color, but pay attention – nuts will burn easily. Let cool a little.

2.	Place the nuts in a clean kitchen towel and rub so that some of the shells come off. The shells which are still stuck can stay there.

3.	Mix all the ingredients in a blender or a food processor to desired consistency. The longer you mix, the smoother it will be.

o) Cinnamon Apples with Vanilla Sauce

Ingredients:

Vanilla sauce

- 8 tablespoons heavy whipping cream
- ½ teaspoon vanilla extract
- 1 star anise (optional)
- 2 tablespoons butter
- 1 egg yolk
- 2 cups heavy whipping cream

Cinnamon apples

- 3 tablespoons butter
- 3 apples, preferably a type that is firm and tart, for example Gravensteiner or Granny Smith
- 1 teaspoon ground cinnamon

Instructions:

1.	Bring the first measurement of heavy whipping cream (1/2 cup), butter, vanilla and optional star anise to a boil in a small saucepan. Lower the heat and let simmer for 5 minutes or more until the sauce turns creamy.

2.   Remove from the heat and remove the star anise. Add the yolk while whisking vigorously. Place in a cool place and let cool completely. This far you can prepare the day before.

3.   Whisk the second measurement of heavy whipping cream (2 cups) in a bowl and mix into the cold cream.

4.   Place in the refrigerator for another 30 minutes or more. You can place them in dessert bowls to make the vanilla sauce thicken up faster.

5.   Wash the apples and peel them if you want to but there's really no need for that. The peel adds color, flavor and texture.

6.   Core the apple and slice thinly. Heat the butter in a frying pan and brown the slices golden. Add cinnamon towards the end.

p) Low-Carb Trifle

Ingredients:

- 1 ripe avocado
- ½ ripe banana
- ¾ cup coconut cream*
- 1 tablespoon lime juice
- 1 pinch limes, only the zest
- 1 tablespoon vanilla extract
- 3½ oz. fresh raspberries
- 2 oz. pecan nuts, preferably roasted

Instructions:

1. Mix together avocado, banana, coconut cream and half of the vanilla. Mix the berries and the rest of the vanilla separately.

2. Fill nice glasses or dessert bowls with alternating layers of the two mixtures.

3. Top with roasted nuts and serve as a dessert.

* You'll find coconut cream next to the regular coconut milk in the grocery store. You can also buy coconut milk and discard the water. Go with the consistency that works for you.

q) Low-Carb Chocolate and Hazelnut Spread

Ingredients:

- 1/3 lb. hazelnuts
- 31/3 tablespoons coconut oil
- 1 oz. butter
- 1 – 2 tablespoons cocoa powder
- 1 teaspoon vanilla extract

Instructions:

1. Roast the hazelnuts in a dry and hot frying pan until they turn a nice color, but pay attention – nuts will burn easily. Let cool a little.

2. Place the nuts in a clean kitchen towel and rub so that some of the shells come off. The shells which are still stuck can stay there.

3. Mix all the ingredients in a blender or a food processor to desired consistency. The longer you mix, the smoother it will be.

r) Microwave Tiramisu

Ingredients:

- 1 tbsp. Erythritol or any sweetener of choice
- ½ tsp. of LC sweet brown sugar without the carbs, you can omit this if you want
- 1 tbsp. of unsalted soften butter
- 3 tbsp. of almond flour (Honeyville brand)
- 2 tbsp. of vanilla whey protein powder
- ¼ tsp. of baking powder
- 1 tbsp. of almond milk
- 2 tbsp. of beaten egg or egg whites

Coffee mixture

- 1 tbsp. of instant coffee
- 2 tbsp. of water

Filling

- 2 oz. cream cheese
- 2 tbsp. whipped cream or heavy cream
- 1 tsp. of Erythritol

Garnish

- 1 tsp. unsweetened cocoa powder
- 1 tsp. of unsweetened grated chocolate

Instructions

1. Cake mixture

2.   First, mix together the sweetener and the softened butter

3.   Next, mix in the rest of the ingredients

4.   Divide into 2 ramekins

5.   Wait a minute for baking powder to activate

6.   Microwave for 1 minute

7.   Filling

8.   Melt cream cheese in microwave for 30 seconds and mix in cream and sweetener.

9.   To Assemble

10.   Cut cake in half

11.   Dip 2 pieces of cake into coffee mixture

12.   Layer the cake with the filling and sprinkle with cocoa and grated chocolate.

Conclusion

In case you're searching for the next action in your dietary experimentation then ketosis is the route forward – or in case you're aspiring to shed pounds, or enhance your cognition.

It's difficult to trust that something as basic as a particularly composed eating regimen can have such a large number of advantages, without any drawbacks. Our predecessors developed with a ketogenic eating routine, and we are deeply rooted in ketosis. Perhaps it works so well since that is how our bodies are developmentally intended to work?

We are however much obliged to you for reading this book. We trust that you have found that it is a simple prologue to the ketogenic diet and we trust that you are propelled to roll out an improvement in your life beginning today.

All that is left is for you to begin and here we encourage you, don't hold up too long-this is not something that ought to be postponed until after the end of the week or until Monday. Begin today in the event that you can – in any event, get out the restricted food from your basic cupboard.

The Ketogenic Diet is a healthful device that can be utilized to drive a caloric shortage in individuals who find the dietary system pleasing and executable.

It doesn't appear to pass on magical weight reduction properties yet it can be utilized as a part of particular settings for fat loss more adequately when it brings about higher adherence. See it as an instrument; utilize it in the correct circumstances!

We wish you the absolute best going ahead. We earnestly trust that you get as much advantage from the ketogenic diet like other individuals have.